SAFER MEDICINE

Mayer Eisenstein, M.D., J.D., M.P.H.

Safer Medicine
Mayer Eisenstein, M.D., J.D., M.P.H.

Published by CMI Press
http://www.homefirst.com

ISBN 0-9670444-1-3 $16.95

Text copyright © 2000 Mayer Eisenstein

Printed in the United States of America

THE 10 GREATEST SETBACKS IN 20TH CENTURY MEDICINE

1. Hospital Birth
2. Routine Birth Interventions (Electronic Fetal Monitoring; Ultrasound; Episiotomy; etc.)
3. Bottle Feeding (Cow's Milk Labeled as Formula)
4. Vaccinations (routine)
5. Antibiotic Abuse
6. The Pill
7. Ritalin
8. Hormone Replacement Therapy (*synthetic*)
9. High Carbohydrate Diets
10. Low Fat Diets

Dr. Eisenstein's favorite aphorisms:

1. Primum Non Nocere - Above all do no harm - Hippocrates

2. Doctors make excellent diagnoses but very poor treatment plans.

3. You must weight the benefits vs. the risks before beginning any treatment plan.

4. Doctors do not let go of one treatment until they find a more dangerous one to replace it.

5. Doctors will scare you of the disease, Mayer Eisenstein, M.D., J.D., M.P.H. will scare you of the treatment.

6. Don't vaccinate before you educate

7. One Grandmother is worth two pediatricians

8. Show me the scientific evidence.

9. Not input measures - but output measures

10. God always forgives - man sometimes forgives - but nature never forgives.

TABLE OF CONTENTS

Preface

We, Americans, worship technology and believe in using the newest, costliest methods available. The internet has made it possible to easily research and evaluate the most current scientific literature. I was privileged to have had Doctors Robert S. Mendelsohn, Herbert Ratner, Gregory White and Beatrice Tucker, as mentors and my goal, in following with their teachings, is to share vital clinical evidence based scientific literature with you and comment on the studies ("M.E. Comments"). Most doctors will try to scare you about different diseases, I will try to scare you about the treatments doctors will try to impose upon you. Through the scientific literature, we see that in most cases, time-honored, low-tech methods, in conjunction with nature are still superior to the high-tech, high intervention approach.

Introduction

What is wrong with this picture? We live in a society where birth takes place in the hospital with induction of labor, routine episiotomy, and cesarean section. Infant formula, antibiotics, and vaccines are given routinely to our children. Young women are on synthetic hormones to prevent pregnancy and then placed on fertility drugs to achieve pregnancy. Our children are medicated in order to learn in school. As we approach menopause we are shifted to another synthetic hormone to prevent symptoms of premeno-pause and menopause. All along our population is diet conscious, yet growing heavier and heavier.

This "modern" medical care has produced a country (America) which ranks 20th, among the top 20 industrial nations with regard to infant and maternal mortality, in spite of spending more money on medical care than any other country in the world.

Have physicians lost their perspective? Don't the scientific studies point to a different direction. The scientific, evidenced based, studies show that birth should take place at home, women should breastfeed, vaccines should be questioned, antibiotics are over prescribed, the Pill is unavoidably dangerous, Ritalin is abused, Hormone Replacement Therapy is dangerous and high carbohydrate/low fat diets are causing obesity. Why are physicians not following the evidence?

I Think - Therefore I Believe

Physicians' attitudes towards medical procedures and treatments have been greatly influenced by their belief systems. If a physician believes something is right, all the scientific studies will not sway his/her thinking. When obstetricians were surveyed with a hypothetical question, "If it is proven that it is 100% safe to deliver a baby vaginally after a previously cesarean section what would you do?" 80% answered they would still do another cesarean section. When questioned about their response, even though the hypothesis stated that it is 100% safe to deliver vaginally after cesarean, their answer was "I do not believe that it is possible." A similar survey was conducted regarding episiotomy. The hypothesis given is that episiotomy is proven to be 100% unnecessary. 80% of physicians surveyed responded they would still perform episiotomies because they believed that episiotomies are necessary.

I was very bothered by these studies because the implication is that even if we conduct definitive scientific studies and even if the results of these studies confirmed my hypothesis, 100% on the safety of home birth, infant feeding, and the dangers of the Pill, HRT, etc. there would be no change in physician behavior.

I asked a theologian, "Why would learned professional physicians not practice medicine in accord with the evidence based scientific studies?" He was not surprised by the findings that I presented to him. He related to me a similar study that he had read. A hypothetical question was posed to people. "If you had the following two choices in life...

1) you and your family would be financially poor all your life, but happy every minute of your life, or

2) you and your family would be financially wealthy all your life, but depressed every minute. You would not be able to change either scenario regardless what you did". Which option would you choose? 80% of the people surveyed chose option 2 - the money. When asked why, they said because I could not believe that with all the money in the world I would not be happy. "You see," the theologian said to me, "Attitudes and beliefs, many times, supercede reality." My belief is that if myths can destroy reality why not make reality destroy the myth? We are facing a very difficult situation in medicine. I am bringing my arguments directly to you the individual who is affected by these procedures, pills, vaccines, etc. in order to give you the ability to say "No" to many unscientific medical procedures. Is the answer to abandon modern medicine? NO, the answer is for medicine to follow the results of the scientific studies which have already been conducted.

Chapter I

Why Home Birth

---

*"Never does nature say one thing
and wisdom another."*
— *Decimus Juniaus Juvenal, Satires*

The safety of home birth, which is something I have always believed on an intuitive level, is explainable through statistical data. I have been looking for years for some way to explain that special edge which home birth mothers have over their hospital birth counterparts.

The answer came one Sunday afternoon, while I was watching a football game on television. The commentator said the home team will win because they have the "HOME COURT ADVANTAGE".

I had heard this expression many times and all of a sudden I said, "that's right! **Home birth has the home court advantage!"**

The expression "home birth advantage" puts into words something I have struggled for years to explain about my home birth practice. Through twenty seven years and 14,000 home deliveries, one of the most recurring questions asked of me continues to be, "What makes home birth safe?"

I don't think the poor hospital statistics mean we have incompetent doctors and nurses in our hospitals. In fact, we have some of the finest doctors in the world. However, our doctors and nurses working in the hospitals lose one very strong advantage — the home court advantage.

Can Hospitals be Made Safe for Birth?

Could the hospital be changed and somehow become as safe as home for laboring women? The answer is "No." There is something about just walking into a hospital that changes the dynamics of labor. The length of labor is significantly increased in the hospital. If you put any woman in the hospital, her labor will slow down or stop because her hormonal balance changes. Her energies have to go into dealing with her strange surroundings, not into the birth itself.

When the mother has been in labor for a "reasonable" amount of time at the hospital without delivering, the doctors believe they must now "actively manage" the labor. They do not realize that the hospital setting is the cause of this problem. They will not believe that this wouldn't have happened at home.

Many "routine interventions" such as drugs, intravenous fluids, electronic monitoring and forceps occur during the hours of labor that wouldn't have existed at home. Hospitals that allow you to labor naturally for the first ten hours won't allow you to labor naturally for the next ten hours. At home these next ten are spent getting to know the already delivered baby, not trying to push the baby out. In other words, the hospital environment creates many of the problems of labor and then obstetricians have to try to solve them.

Home births occur before the miserable second half of hospital labor has a chance to start. Home births occur before problems happen. If women knew that most of them could have half as much labor and no complications, they would all be choosing home birth!

Prior to this century, birth always took place in the comfort of home with close friends and family surrounding the mother. Giving birth requires privacy and intimacy. Birth is a very sexual and personal experience. A warm, intimate and supportive environment allows us to function as we were intended.

Is Home Birth
Scientifically Sound?

Home birth doctors, often get labeled as unscientific. They are pictured as "hippie leftovers" from the 1960's or practitioners of some dangerous cult which tortures women and babies. Home birth has even been called the earliest form of child abuse. I guess, there was a lot of abuse going on before the 1940's when birth made it's move to hospitals.

Modern technology is being applied inappropriately during most hospital births, producing disastrously long labors, birth accidents and poor bonding opportunities for mothers and babies. This is unacceptable.

Another frequently asked question regarding the safety of home birth is, "What does the medical establishment think of having babies at home?"

I can only answer that question by citing the scientific literature of the medical establishment. Traditional establishment medical journals reinforce, over and over again, the safety of physician attended home birth. It is the obstetricians who are not following the recommendations of their own professional journals.

In the scientific literature one learns that for the low-risk pregnant woman, there is no need for electronic fetal monitors, IV fluids, ultrasound, episiotomies or the traditional position for hospital labor and delivery, namely, the woman flat on her back in bed. Over 90% of all pregnant women are low risk and they are all being treated as high-risk by modern obstetricians.

In obstetrical journals and other current publications there were over 160 articles supporting the findings that a vaginal birth is much safer for someone who has had a previous cesarean section delivery. However, only 20% of women are being given a chance, by their doctors, to have a vaginal delivery after a previous cesarean section.

One more consistently used unnecessary intervention is the routine use of ultrasound. Ultrasound waves actually raise the temperature of the amniotic fluid which surrounds the unborn baby. We just don't know the impact of this on such small bodies. This technique should be applied only in cases where a problem is strongly suspected, not to predict delivery dates, not to determine the sex of the baby and certainly not to show the mother a "first picture" of her baby. Nature determines the optimal date for the baby's birthday, not an inaccurate technological device whose results can be off by weeks.

Ultrasound, I believe, will soon be discovered to be as unsafe as x-rays were found to be. Pregnant women were routinely x-rayed in the 1940's. These x-rays resulted in many cases of cancer.

The most important point I can make is that consumers can verify my findings for themselves in medical literature. I would like to let couples know that they can and should research the safety of various tests and explore birthing options for themselves in current obstetrical literature.

Anyone can go online and use the internet to look up topics such as "ultrasound," "episiotomy" or "cesarean section" and find many articles about the proper use of these procedures. You will read scientific evidence which supports the non-interventionist approach.

Home Birth & Emergency Situations

This brings me back to the **Home Court Advantage**. I recently heard an interview with an obstetrician on staff at a teaching hospital who stated that almost every day, at the hospital, there is a birth that starts out absolutely normal then something goes awry. This was his reason why birth has to be in the hospital. Home birth physicians believe just the opposite. Virtually every birth starts out normal and we do everything we can to keep it that way. The over 100 pieces of emergency medical equipment (i.e. I.V. fluids, resuscitation equipment, plasma expanders, drugs and medication, etc.), which are brought to the home, by the home birth physician, enable the home birth physician to respond to medical needs of labor. Should an emergency arise with the laboring woman, i.e. the need for blood replacement (in 27 years and over 14,000 births, we have administered blood only four times), or emergency cesarean section (less than 10 emergency cesareans in 27 years. The sophisticated transport and communication systems available today virtually equal the speed with which the same arrangements could be made in a hospital. Remember, the hospital cannot perform surgery in the labor room. The American College of Obstetrics and Gynecology finds it within the accepted standard of medical care to perform the cesarean section within one hour after the decision is made. Also, blood is not available in the labor and/or delivery room but the woman must be typed and cross matched again - which virtually equals the time required to transfer the laboring woman and receive the blood replacement.

Women Can Enjoy Giving Birth

Women laboring at home actually enjoy giving birth. The mothers are surrounded by familiar sights, smells, foods, and most importantly by people who care about them. No one has to worry about which unfamiliar people will be walking in or what they will be doing which might alter the progress of labor. Often, after the baby is born, the parents are already talking about having another baby. How often is this heard after a hospital birth?

Modern childbirth classes teach the husband to fight for his wife and baby's best interests during delivery. The husband is always placed in a dilemma at hospital birth. How can he possibly know how to fight against an entire medical staff making recommendations for fetal monitors, drugs, or even cesarean sections? One of the nicest things about home as a birth setting is that husbands don't have to take a defensive position. They don't have to fight to have basic sound scientific technique applied to their wife's labor and delivery. At home everyone's energy can go into the birth, not into a fight about the principles of safe birth.

Prenatal Care in the Homefirst® System

The trust families have in home birth physicians is one that has been earned during the course of prenatal care. Husbands and wives have come to know that their home birth physicians will keep their promises about birth and that whatever decisions are made in labor and delivery are in the best interest of the mother and baby. This is a tremendously comforting feeling both during pregnancy and delivery.

It is the role of home birth physicians to create a caring atmosphere from the beginning of pregnancy, and to help families feel positive about their labor, delivery and, of course, about the expected child. We share in the families' feelings of excitement about birth and we are delighted in our role of helping to bring new life into our expectant families' homes. These shared feelings become the prime motivation for the continued good health of the pregnant mother.

At prenatal visits it is our desire to establish trust and confidence between the home birth physician and the expectant family. This is the kind of trust patients used to place in the family's general practitioner, who knew them well and often treated them in their own homes.

This type of trust maintains health in a way **routine** prenatal tests and procedures never could. It also makes the future labor and delivery go faster and smoother because the family knows there is nothing unexpected about the home birth physicians and their methods. As the home birth physicians promise - no unnecessary interventions are done in the family's home. The physician will arrive with the primary goal of maintaining a safe and comfortable atmosphere for the laboring mother. This establishes an emotional wellness within the family most conducive to safe birth.

A grandfather who was attending one of my Sunday night home birth seminars expressed it better than I ever could. He was there with his two daughters, both of them pregnant. One of his daughters had had a child at home previously and now both daughters were scheduled for home births.

Their father got up and said, "I love what Homefirst® Health Services is doing. I believe that the emotional wellness of home birth that you talk about is the same as love. It is the outpouring of the love your doctors and nurses have for their patients that makes a difference. That love causes the "release of medicines" in the laboring women that science hasn't even found yet — medicines that make things go well at home. We have to look to "new," but really ancient, birthing techniques in our country to return America to being a safe birthing place. It is time to take a look at doctors like myself and those in my practice — home birth physicians — and our implementation of scientific techniques. It is time to reexamine our own culture's birthing history.

Chicago is rich in physician home birth history. The physicians from The Chicago Maternity Center served the city from 1895 through 1972 delivering over 100,000 babies at home, with a safety record unsurpassed in America. It is time to examine the techniques of countries which have excellent safety records for delivery of infants and the health of mothers and babies. Interestingly enough, countries at the top of the list are those with a large home birth component.

Who Has Home Births
These Days

In the 1990's, an interesting aspect of the home birth trend is that middle and upper class families are opting for home birth. Well-read and well-educated families are looking into our "new" idea of home birth because they are discovering that it is safer. They are disturbed by what modern obstetrics has been doing to women and babies and are learning about alternatives for themselves. Anyone who does some investigating of his/her own does not want to be a part of the alarming statistics related to hospital birth.

Most home birth parents are college graduates. Many of the mothers are nurses and many of the fathers are employed in high tech positions. They are people who understand the importance and safety of the natural birth process. They realize that giving birth is hard work, best performed in accordance with the laws of nature. They believe that for this reason alone, birth must happen at home. If it were simply a mechanical process, then the hospital would be a good enough alternative location.

Scientific Studies on
Home Birth

Professor Tew, in an article in *J R Coll Gen Pract* 1985;35(277):390-394, titled **Scientific Studies on Home Birth** discusses the place of birth with regard to perinatal mortality. She writes that:

"Using the raw PMRs (PMR = Perinatal mortality rate: usually defined as the number of deaths occurring between 28 weeks gestation and 7 days after birth divided by the number of stillborn infants of at least 28 weeks gestation plus all liveborn infants in the same population regardless of gestational age; usually expressed per 1000) from a 1970 British national survey, the hospital PMR was 27.8 per 1000 births versus 5.4 per 1000 for home births/general practitioner units (GPU). This was not because hospitals handled more high-risk births. When PMRs were standardized based on age, parity, hypertension/toxemia, prenatal risk prediction score, method of delivery, and birth weight, adjusted hospital PMRs for each category ranged from 22.7 per 1000 to 27.8 per 1000 while home birth/CPU rates ranged from 5.4 per 1000 to 10.5 per 1000."

PMR

Perinatal Mortality Rate

	Home	Hospital
All Births	5.4 (per 1,000 births)	27.8 (per 1,000 births)
High Risk	15.5 (per 1,000 births)	--
Low Risk	--	17.9 (per 1,000 births)

"The 1970 survey assigned a prenatal risk score to predict the likelihood of problems during labor. When PMRs for hospital versus home/GPU for the same level of risk (very low, low, moderate, high, very high) are compared, the hospital PMR was lower only at the very highest risk level. All differences, except in the "very high risk" category, were significant. The PMR for high-risk births in home/GPUs (15.5/1000) was slightly lower than that for low-risk births in the hospital (17.9/1000). Moreover, the PMRs in home/GPUs for very low, low, and moderate risk births were all similar, but hospital PMRs increased twofold between categories, **which suggests that hospital labor management actually intensified risks**.

The percentage of infants born with breathing difficulties (9.3% versus 3.3%), the death rate associated with breathing difficulties (0.94% versus 0.19%), and the transfer rate to neonatal intensive care units for infants with breathing problems who survived six hours (62.0% versus 26.2%) were all higher in the hospital (all p <0.001), further evidence that hospital interventions do not avert poor outcomes.

Although no national study has been undertaken since, smaller studies confirm that increasing use of hospital confinement is not the reason for the overall drop in PMR since 1970. In fact, those years when the proportional increase in hospital births was greatest were the years when the PMR declined least and vice versa."

M.E. Comments:

Tew's study shows that the PMR for high risk at home (15.5) was slightly lower than the PMR for low risk in the hospital (17.9) which means it was safer to deliver a high risk baby at home than a low risk baby in the hospital. When you look at the overall PMR it is 500% more dangerous to deliver in the hospital. Why would anyone have their baby in the hospital after reading this study?

೮ଛ೮ଛ

In the medical journal, *Med J Aust* 1988;149(6):296-302, Dr. KA Howe discusses **Home Births in South-West Australia.**

"The outcomes of 165 home births between 1983 and 1986 from the practices of all six midwives located in southwest Australia are reviewed. Sixteen percent were transferred to the hospital for birth complications. The cesarean rate was 1.2%, the assisted vaginal delivery rate was 4.8%, the induction rate was 0%, and the augmentation rate was 3%. One baby died of congenital anomalies, and another had good Apgar scores but then developed respiratory difficulties. The baby was transported to the hospital and made a spontaneous recovery.

It is interesting to speculate on the reasons for such consistently favourable results in studies on home birth. One hypothesis is that the common obstetric interventions at best do not improve outcome and at worst are hazardous; this implies that their use should be reduced drastically. Alternatively, the intervention rates may be appropriate for the hospital population but are not necessary for women who are giving birth at home; this implies that one or more factors are operating at home to facilitate the progress of normal labor. Suggested factors are: the surroundings at home are more relaxed . . . ; the relationship between the home-birth midwife and the patient is much stronger and therefore perhaps more "therapeutic". . . ; and the home-birth mothers are more strongly motivated than are their hospital counterparts, and this motivation is a strong positive factor in terms of outcome."

M.E. Comments:

Howe's study confirms the established concept that obstetrical intervention takes place far less in the home than in the hospital. As far back as 1933, in a major study entitled "Maternal Mortality in New York City, the New York Academy of Medicine Committee of Public Health under the direction of Ransom S. Hooker, M.D., came to the following conclusion "There can be little doubt that the ready facilities of a hospital tend to casual operative interference, while conditions at home preclude operation unless there are urgent indications... The great increase in hospitalization of the normal parturient has failed to bring the hoped for reduction in puerperal morbidity and mortality... It would seem that the present attitude toward home confinement requires reexamination, and a program looking toward an increase in the practice of domiciliary [home] obstetrics deserves careful investigation." Almost 70 years later the same conclusions seem to be true.

ೞೞೞೞ

In 1996 *the **British Medical Journal**,* No. 7068 Volume 313, Saturday 23 November 1996 published four studies on the safety of home birth, accompanied by an excellent editorial by Dr. Nachel P Springer, Professor Department of

General Practice, Leiden University, Leiden, Netherlands and Dr. Chris Van Weel, Professor Department of General Practice & Social Medicine. These studies added to the evidence that in selected women, with adequate infrastructure and support, home birth is safe. Dr. Springer writes...

"Birth is an event of great importance in family life. Although pregnancy and delivery are, under healthy conditions, normal social and physiological processes, childbirth has become hospital centered in most industrialized countries. The assumption is that hospital based deliveries are safer for mother and child. Yet, the Cumberlege report sees home birth as a real option, and the wishes of women to have home births must be viewed in that light. A randomized controlled trial would help to resolve the controversy over the relative safety of home and hospital birth, but conditions for a "fair" trial are difficult to achieve. Such a study would require large numbers because of the low frequency of adverse events, and the necessary environment of experienced home deliveries has virtually disappeared. In the absence of a randomized trial, observational studies are welcome, and this week's BMJ carries four papers reporting on the safety, professional support, and patient satisfaction of home births.

The first of these, from the Northern region's perinatal mortality survey, reports 134 perinatal losses in 3466 births outside the hospital, about four times the number of losses in hospital births. At first sight this seems to endorse the view that hospital is the safest place to deliver. But 97% (131) of these perinatal deaths at home were recorded in women who were actually booked for a hospital delivery or had no prearranged plan for delivery. **The perinatal outcome in planned home births was better than for all women giving birth in the region** - a result in line with Swiss and Dutch findings also reported in this week's BMJ. This supports the safety of home birth provided it is offered to women at low risk of obstetric complications. Most perinatal deaths occur in women with health or obstetric problems that existed before or developed during pregnancy, and these women can be identified and referred before the onset of labour."

M.E. Comments: In 1992, the British House of Commons Select Committee on Maternity Services (Winterton Report) concluded, "There is no convincing or compelling evidence that hospitals give a better guarantee of the safety of the majority of mother and babies. It is possible that the contrary may be the case." The above 1996, British Medical Journal, editorial, which reviewed four scientific papers reporting on the safety, professional support and the patient satisfaction with home birth came to the same conclusion regarding the safety of home birth.

ങ⊰ങ⊰ങ⊰

REFERENCES

Acheson L S, Harris S E, Zyzanski S J. "Patient selection and outcomes for out-of-hospital births in one family practice." Journal of Family Practice 1990;31: 128-36.

Ackermann-Liebrich U, Voegli T, Guenther-Witt K, Kunz I, Zullig M, Schindler C, et al. "Home versus hospital deliveries: a prospective study on matched pairs." British Medical Journal 1996;313:1313-8.

Cunningham D J. "Experiences of Australian mothers who gave birth either at home, or in hospital labour wards." Soc Sci Med 1993 ;36:473-83.

Davies J, Hey E, Reid W, Young G. "Prospective regional study of planned home birth." British Medical Journal, 1996;313: 1302-5.

Department of Health Expert Maternity Group. "Changing childbirth." 1. The Cumberledge report. London: **HMSO**, 1993.

"Education and debate. Should there be a trial of home versus hospital delivery in the United Kingdom." British Medical Journal, 1996;312:753-7.

Eisenstein, Mayer, Home Birth Advantage, CMI Press, 2000.

Homefirst® Web Page at http://www.homefirst.com

Springer M E. "Quality of obstetric performance of general
    practitioners" [Kwaliteit van het verloskundig handelen
    van huisartsen] [thesis]. Leiden: Leiden University,
    1991. (English summary.)

Tew, Marjorie, Safer Childbirth?, 1998, FA Books.

Tew, Marjorie, "Do Obstetrical Intranatal Interventions Make
    Birth Safe?," British Journal of Obstetrics and
    Gynecology, July, 1986.

"The Northern Region's Perinatal Mortality Survey
    Coordinating Group. Perinatal loss in planned and
    unplanned home birth." British Medical
    Journal,1996;313: 1306-9.

Wiegers T A, Keirse M J N C, van der Zee J, Berghs G A H.
    "Outcome of planned home and planned hospital births
    in low risk pregnancies in the Netherlands." British
    Medical Journal, 1996;313:1309-13.

Chapter II

Exposing the
Cesarean Myth

*"It is dangerous to be right on a subject
on which the established authorities
are wrong"*
Voltaire

The maternal mortality from cesarean section is 10 to 20 times greater than from a vaginal delivery. Despite all of the recent scientific evidence, showing that the c-section rate is too high [25-30% in United States hospitals versus less than 5% by home birth physicians], the rate continues to climb. The countries which have the lowest cesarean section rates, (i.e. Norway, Denmark, Sweden, Holland, Japan, etc.) also have the lowest infant and maternal mortality rates in the world.

The mantra "once a cesarean always a cesarean" is being used by doctors today despite all the lip service that they give to vaginal birth after cesarean. In 1987, less than 2% of women in this country who had previous cesareans actually delivered their next babies vaginally. We, at Homefirst® Health Services, have been privileged to successfully deliver over 1,000 HBAC (home birth after cesarean) babies since 1988, with a vaginal success rate of 90%. Success cannot only be measured by vaginal birth, the other 10% were just as successful, even though delivered by cesarean. The success of our HBAC program rests with the skills of our physicians and nurses, as well as a philosophy that unnecessary medical interventions, (i.e. electronic fetal monitoring, epidural medication, routine cesarean section for breech and twin deliveries, etc.) at the time of delivery are some of the major causes of unnecessary cesarean sections.

We have reached a time when women must become educated about cesarean section prevention long before the birth of their first child. In the new millennium unnecessary cesarean sections are analogous to environmental hazards. In order to be protected from radon gas in your home, for example, you must be informed of the dangers and take the appropriate action to protect your family. The same is true of c-section surgery. Education is the best prevention method families have from this hazardous surgery.

I use the term hazardous because it is. In 1987, a 14-state survey from the Center for Disease Control indicated that babies over 1500 grams (3.1 pounds) are more likely to die if born by cesarean section than if born vaginally. The risk to the mother is many times greater when surgery is performed. Recovery from c-section surgery is painful and slow, leaving the mother with psychological, as well as abdominal scars.

Our goal as doctors must be to deliver healthy babies to healthy mothers. Doctors must aim to make America the safest country in the world in which to have a baby. We now rank 20th among the top 20 industrialized nations for infant and maternal mortality. It is unethical and unthinkable that any doctor would be performing unnecessary c-sections, but it is happening with too great frequency today.

Ten years ago doctors were delivering babies by cesarean section at a 6% rate, eight years ago at a 10% rate, five years ago at a 15% rate and three years ago at a 20% rate. In 1987, a jump in the rate to between 25% and 30% occurred, translating into one million plus Americans having c-section deliveries in that year. Doctors, supposedly, have increased their c-section rates in the U.S. as one means of decreasing our infant mortality, but the infant mortality rate has risen dramatically.

Why So Many Cesarean Sections?

About one in four women is now having this surgery for the delivery of her child. In Illinois, according to a *Chicago Sun Times* report of March 16, 1988, there was a 10% increase in cesarean sections. Blue Cross/Blue Shield of Illinois is urging hospitals to slow the growing rate of surgical deliveries. The National Institutes of Health (N.I.H.), a neutral body, likewise says that there are too many cesareans being performed. N.I.H. believes that obstetricians aren't willing to make changes to improve this statistic.

These findings really hit home for my staff and myself when our practice had a booth at a baby fair in Chicago a few years ago. We were at the fair to explain the home birth option to those who didn't realize that babies could be safely born at home. However, over the course of the fair, about 1,000 women who had previously had cesarean section deliveries stopped by our booth to talk.

Many of them were pregnant again and returning to their same obstetricians for planned, repeat c-section deliveries. They were feeling their bodies had failed them and were wondering if surgery would really be necessary the second time. We were shocked and realized we had to do something to help these women. With the c-section rate rising as it is, by the turn of the century all women will be having c-sections, a ridiculous but plausible thought. We felt we had to intervene to change this statistic. Since our own c-section rate was about 4% we felt there must be something we could do to provide safer deliveries for so many women fearing unnecessary repeat surgery for the births of their next infants. Our research led us to some very positive conclusions. Statistics collected by my Homefirst® medical staff revealed that 90-92% of all pregnant women should be able to deliver their babies without any medical intervention at all. It was puzzling to me why so many doctors were choosing a measure so drastic as surgery for the delivery of so many babies.

According to the March 16, 1988, *Sun Times* article quoted above ". . .doctors in major teaching hospitals tend to have lower c-section rates because doctors there have a heightened awareness of the overuse of c-sections." This implies that with doctor awareness the rate could be lowered. This article was clearly saying that doctors are the cause of so many c-sections.

Everyone knows why Blue Cross/Blue Shield is mentioned in the article as being interested in lowering the c-section rate. Theirs is the financial interest of an insurer who has to pay out much more per birth on a c-section delivery. Currently c-sections average about $3,000 more per birth than a natural delivery. Blue Cross/Blue Shield's research was saying the same thing to hospitals — there are too many unnecessary c-sections. Dr. Norbert Gleicher, former Director of Maternal-Fetal Medicine at Mount Sinai Medical Center in Chicago is quoted in the article as being concerned that unnecessary c-sections expose women to risks of infection and other problems. He believes the bottom line is going to have to be financial. "Scientific data and education haven't been enough to get doctors to lower the rates. . . . If insurers want to reduce the c-section rate, they will have to give doctors and hospitals a financial incentive for vaginal deliveries." This certainly implies that doctors are doing c-sections for the added income which this surgery generates.

So here too, with the high c-section rate we see unscientific medicine being practiced in yet another area. Doctors continue to disregard the scientific literature. Why? A misguided sense of security from malpractice lawsuits, additional income, and a false assumption that their patients have had a safer delivery. These are powerful obstacles to hurdle if you are an uninformed patient. The less informed patient, the greater the chances of a cesarean section. It has become imperative to be an educated pregnant woman in order to have the safe delivery of a baby today.

Doctors' Myths About Cesarean Section

The doctors in my practice did further research. The reasons for most c-sections were not grounded in good scientific practice, but rather in doctor myths such as, "Once a c-section, always a c-section." A whole body of medical phrases has been invented to justify the surgical delivery of infants. Mothers are being told that: they "failed to progress" in labor; the baby's head was too large for the pelvis; they had a "cephalo-pelvic disproportion"; twins and breech babies must be delivered by c-section, and that vaginal delivery after a previous c-section is dangerous due to the likelihood of "uterine rupture."

These reasons for c-section and repeat c-section surgery are unfounded in most cases. In 1997, c-section surgery was the number one surgical procedure performed in the United States. Over 1,000,000 women had this surgery for delivery of their babies. If an acceptable rate of c-section surgery is 5%, then 850,000 women had unnecessary and dangerous operations.

Women are being deprived of vaginally delivering their babies for reasons other than those stated to them by doctors. Could doctors actually believe that c-sections are safer and easier than natural delivery? This is absurd. It is impossible to comprehend that an ethical practitioner would choose a procedure "safer" for himself and more dangerous for the mother and her baby. Various studies have indicated that c-section delivery is from 8 to 26 times more dangerous than natural delivery. Today's mothers and babies are suffering unnecessarily, and even dying, from cesarean deliveries.

A 1986 publication of the Public Citizen Health Research Group entitled *Unnecessary Cesarean Sections: A Rapidly Growing National Epidemic* states that:

The three most important medical causes contributing to the rapid national increase in c-section rates are:

1) the continued use of the outdated policy of automatic repeat c-section for women who have already had a c-section.
2) the over diagnosis and overuse of c-section for dystocia (or abnormal labor), and
3) the over diagnosis of fetal distress.

These three categories contributed to 93.4% of the increase in national c-section rates from 1980 to 1985.

C-section surgery does have a few benefits for an insecure, fearful or inexperienced doctor. Surgery is quicker than waiting for labor and delivery to happen on its own. It seems safer to the doctor because he/she doesn't have to watch the mother progress through the pains of labor which can be a tremendously lengthy and anxious experience for everyone. Obstetricians who don't understand the scientific principles of labor and delivery might actually believe they are saving mothers from a lot of pain by performing a c-section. We know they **believe** they are saving themselves from potential lawsuits.

But these are incorrect and unethical reasons for performing surgery on any pregnant woman. As one of the new doctors on my staff put it, "We were trained in medical school that a pregnant woman is something to be feared. She is considered ill until she delivers, and the sooner the better."

My staff and I did much investigating of the explanations given to families for their c-section deliveries. We discovered fallacies in all the explanations.

The doctor's myth, "Once a c-section, always a c-section," has never been proven. This statement, first made by an intoxicated physician at a medical meeting, is only espoused by doctors with no understanding of the contractility of the uterus. The uterus is a tremendously strong muscle. It contracts as other muscles do in order to function. Much as the heart muscle contracts to pump blood, the uterine muscle contracts and expands in labor to deliver the baby. A scar on the uterus from a previous c-section negligibly lowers its ability to contract properly. So you might say that for most women the opposite of this myth is true, "Once a c-section, next time a VBAC." Each labor is unique and a doctor is suspect who prejudges the outcome of the next labor after a c-section.

Exposing the Myths

Many women whose obstetricians have scared them with the threat of a repeat c-section ask me how any woman who has had a previous c-section could be a low risk patient in my practice. They have all been labeled by their obstetricians as high risk due to their last deliveries. In reality, provided the woman is in good health, she should be treated no differently from any other pregnant woman. She will become high risk only if doctors use interventionist measures at the time of delivery.

Another doctor's myth, about which women are so frequently warned, is the feared "uterine rupture" which occurs rarely in births subsequent to c-sections. Contrary to the doctor's myth, scientific literature supports the fact that the uterus does not rupture from and has not been weakened by a previous c-section delivery. Two investigators reported, in separate presentations to the American College of Obstetricians and Gynecologists, that they "have been unable to find a single report of a maternal death due to rupture of a low transverse uterine incision in the more than 11,000 trials of labor." This statement was made after reviewing data collected at the University of California, Los Angeles, School of Medicine; Kaiser Permanente Medical Centers and the University of California, Irvine, School of Medicine (as reported in *Family Practice News*, Volume 18, No. 14, July 15--31, 1988). Uterine rupture is just another well-propagated myth.

Then there is the often-used expression, "failure to prog- ress," which leads to surgery. Doctors use this phrase at hospital births for several reasons. They have placed women flat on their backs and on the hospital's timetable for delivery. If progress isn't made in a given amount of time, they prepare for surgical delivery. But "failure to progress" is predictable if a woman is on her back for eight or nine hours and pushing in this very unnatural position.

It becomes a different matter if someone at home, who is not confined to bed during labor, has "failure to progress." The laboring woman has then done everything in her power to deliver in a reasonable amount of time. However, as I have discussed in a previous chapter, timetables for labor get distorted in the hospital. Labor time in the hospital doubles because doctors don't make the best use of that time. Dr. Emanual Friedman of Boston's Beth Israel Hospital and Harvard Medical School has stated that 70% of cesareans for prolonged labor are unnecessary.

Hand in hand with "failure to progress" goes another classical mythical reason for c-section deliveries — CPD — "cephalo-pelvic disproportion." This first myth leads doctors to suspect the second. "Cephalo-pelvic disproportion" means that the baby's head is too large for delivery through the mother's "too small" pelvis. It is easy for doctors to incorrectly conclude that if a woman has "failure to progress," it is because the baby's head is too large for delivery.

In reality, this doesn't happen very often. Nature allows women to grow babies to a size proper for delivery by that individual mother. If this were really a problem occurring frequently in nature all babies born to small women such as Chinese, Thai, and Japanese would be c-section babies. However, in these countries c-sections are rarely performed.

Babies, born at home, to mothers who have had previous c-sections are usually larger than older cesarean-born siblings. These later, natural born babies disprove the disproportion problem, by being larger than their older siblings at birth. Generally, it is improperly used labor time or an unwarranted fear of birth accidents which prompts doctors to write CPD on the mother's chart and prepare her for surgery.

The myth that twins and breech babies must be delivered by surgery is a ridiculous notion also. Doctors have been intervening in these types of births for so long that the skills necessary to deliver multiples have been lost. It is actually a five-year program to train doctors properly to deliver twins and breech babies. However, a new doctor can learn to do a c-section in about 90 days. Preference for the shorter training time and fear of lawsuits, has virtually eradicated all knowledge of natural delivery of these babies from U.S. hospitals.

The Birth of
HBAC

In the past, my staff and I had assisted women in hospitals who were trying to have vaginal births after cesarean (VBAC). We noticed that they succeeded only about 50 to 60% of the time in the hospital. We felt sure that this was due to the foreign environment and that a higher success rate could be achieved at home because women have an easier time delivering at home. It would seem unnecessary to hospitalize these women at all if the scientific literature were correct. All reputable obstetrical literature states that VBAC women are no different from anyone else in labor if they have no other medical complications.

So a plan evolved within my practice during the summer of 1987 to let VBAC women labor at home in the comfort of their own surroundings, with the support of their families and the careful monitoring of the Homefirst® medical staff. The plan was initiated by Dr. Peter S.L. Rosi, one of the Homefirst® senior staff physicians. Dr. Rosi, in addition to being a home birth specialist, is a board certified surgeon. This project became known as HBAC, Home Birth After Cesarean.

We chuckle to ourselves when we look back to those first HBAC births. In the name of safety, two doctors and two nurses from the practice were sent to these laboring women's homes. Of course it soon became apparent, due to careful prenatal screening, that there was no need to provide more medical support than any other home birth mother receives. Eighty-seven percent of this pilot group had their babies at home with no complications or need for intervention.

This program has been a tremendous success. Now potential HBAC mothers attend our childbirth classes alongside those who have had successful home births in the past. There is no reason to treat HBAC women differently from other pregnant women, unless new indications point to a possible problem.

We do have a few additional recommendations for HBAC mothers. We tell them not to return to the doctor who performed the first c-section surgery. That doctor will view the returning woman as trouble. That doctor will, chances are, have his or her mind made up in advance that there will be complications.

We also suggest that HBAC couples connect with a VBAC Support Group to increase their chances of having a vaginal birth. Jane, leader of a VBAC Support Group in Chicago says, "If women attend our sessions, they increase their chances of having a vaginal birth. We help them lay to rest the fear of uterine rupture and try to connect them with doctors who will give them a fair chance at a vaginal delivery. C-section mothers have been stripped of all confidence in their bodies' ability to give birth and they need the support of other women who have "been there" to regain their confidence. It is a lack of education and the feeling that the doctor is always right that leads to many c-sections. This is what we work on. Being at home for the next birth and knowing how to give birth helps so much!"

Too Many
Cesarean Sections

Dr. Rydhstrom, author of the article *"The Impact of Cesarean Section in Relation to Fetal Presentation"* which appeared in *American Journal of Obstetrics and Gynecology*, 163:528-533, 1990, concluded that cesarean section appears to have little impact on fetal outcome for low birth weight twins, even after considering fetal presentation. In a review of this article Peter Boylan, M.D., Master, National Maternity Hospital, Dublin, Ireland, stated:

"This is an important study that fails to support the liberal use of cesarean sections for twins with a birth weight of less than 1,500 grams. This is particularly interesting in view of the fact that no advantage was found even for twins where the baby was presenting by the breech. The study is also interesting in that there was no decline in incidents of cerebral palsy during the decade examined, despite a tenfold increase in cesarean section. The study provides support for those who wish to continue with a conservative approach toward the care of women and babies around the time of delivery. **It is becoming more apparent with the passage of time that Cesarean birth rates may be used as an index of the quality of**

**care given to women, and that a low Cesarean
section rate equates with a high standard of care."**

M.E. Comments:

*The findings by Dr. Rydhstrom that cesarean section is
unwarranted for low birth weight twins and Dr. Boylan's
commentary that high cesarean section is an index of low
quality in obstetrical care, will hopefully change physicians'
attitudes toward cesarean section.*

ଔଔଔଔ

On May 22, 1994, "The New York Times National"
Washington, May 21 (AP), wrote...

"420,000 C-Sections a Year Are Called Unneeded
Each year, some 420,000 deliveries of babies in the
United States use unnecessary Caesarean sections, a
consumer group has contended.

The highest rates are in the South and at large for-
profit hospitals, the Public Citizen Health Research
Group said on Wednesday. But it said that surgical
deliveries were dropping slightly and that more women
were delivering babies vaginally after previous
Caesareans.

The group examined birth records that show 22.6
percent of the nearly four million births in 1992 were
Caesareans, making the operation the most common

major surgery performed in this country. That is down slightly from a 22.7 percent Caesarean rate in 1991. Caesareans, commonly known as C-sections, often save the lives of babies during long or complicated labor, but the surgery can also endanger the mother. In 1970, Caesareans were used in 5.5 percent of births, but they skyrocketed to 24.7 percent in 1988.

Consumer advocates say only 12 percent of births should be by Caesarean, and the Centers for Disease Control and Prevention advocates a rate of no higher than 15 percent.

Using the 12 percent mark, the consumer group said, about 420,000 unnecessary C-sections were performed at a cost of $1.3 billion in 1992 the latest year for which data are available...."

ಐಐಐಐ

In 1996, the Institute for Healthcare Improvement sponsored a collaborative program in an attempt to educate doctors on how to lower the cesarean section rate. Miriam E. Tucker, *Staff Writer* for FAMILY PRACTICE NEWS in her column Women's Health, January 1, 1996, writes,

"... The collaborative (program) was sponsored by the Institute for Healthcare Improvement (IHI), Boston, a nonprofit organization that aims to improve health care delivery.

At a meeting on reducing cesarean section rates sponsored by IHI (14 months after the collaborative began), participants shared information about what worked and what didn't.

Dr. Bruce Flamm, who chaired the congress, noted that while both the U.S. Public Health Service and the World Health Organization have set a cesarean section rate target of 15% by the year 2000, not everyone shares that goal.

'If you agree that the current 23% rate should be reduced, there are safe ways to do it,' Dr. Flamm, area research chairman and practicing OB/GYN. at Kaiser Permanente, Riverside, California....

Ways to Reduce Your Cesarean Section Rate

The following are "change concepts", that organizations in the multi center collaborative were encouraged to follow to reduce unnecessary cesarean sections.

'The science is not new, but the framework is,' *collaborative chairman Bruce Flamm said. "The more you do, the better, but you don't have to do everything. Pick one small change you can implement by next Tuesday," he advised....*

<u>Avoid unnecessary interventions</u>

Interventions such as artificial rupture of membranes or induction often result in imposition of time limits and cesarean section if the baby isn't delivered within that time. Instead, do only what's absolutely necessary and no more.

- Use expectant management for spontaneous rupture of membranes rather than immediate routine induction.
- Do not routinely induce for postdates prior to 42 weeks' gestation unless there are other indications.
- Avoid estimating fetal weight by ultrasound after 36 weeks.
- Consider using intermittent monitoring or auscultation instead of routine electronic fetal monitoring.
- Give patients a "due week," rather than a "due date."...

Provide effective labor support

It's important to treat labor as a natural, physiologic process and not to over rely on technology,

- Provide one-to-one psychological support through nurses or doulas.
- Give oral hydration to assist patients in their physical efforts and reduce the impression that they're being prepared for surgery

- Turn off central fetal monitors except at change of shift; have nurses spend more time talking to the patients.

Manage high-risk conditions

Conditions such as herpes simplex virus, twin pregnancies, and breech presentation should not be seen as automatic indications for cesarean delivery.

- Develop and use criteria for vaginal delivery in patients with genital herpes.
- Develop and use criteria for trial of labor in twin gestations, based on gestational age and fetal positions.
- Use external cephalic version at 37 weeks' gestation for breech presentation.

To Avoid Unnecessary Repeat Cesarean Sections:
Plan a trial of labor

- Use American College of Obstetricians and Gynecologists guidelines or other criteria for elective repeat cesarean section and use these to develop vaginal birth after cesarean (VBAC) guidelines. Circulate to all staff.
- Review all repeat cesarean sections to ascertain medical necessity either as a posthoc review process or as precertification."

M.E. Comments:

Dr. Bruce Flamm has been a pioneer in teaching the concept of the safety of vaginal birth after cesarean section. As the Chairman of the Collaborative Committee to Lower the Cesarean Section Rate, he once again shows his true dedication to evidence based medicine. The over 1,000 "hbac" deliveries (home birth after cesarean) that Homefirst® Health Services has participated in is also further support for the teaching of Dr. Flamm that "once a cesarean does not mean always a cesarean".

Another way to lower the cesarean section is to reduce the use of epidural anesthesia during a first stage of labor. Dr. Lieberman, in a meeting of the Society for Perinatal Obstetricians, presented a study which showed that the use of epidural anaesthesia during the first stage of labor may at least triple the chance that women will deliver their babies by cesarean section and that women who receive epidurals before 5 cm dilation were 5.4 times as likely to deliver by cesarean section. "Medical Tribune *for the Obstetrician & Gynecologist*", February 16, 1995 - Volume 2, Number 4.

REFERENCES

"420,000 C-Sections a Year Are Called Unneeded" *The New York Times National Sunday,* May 22, 1994

"Comparisons of National Cesarean-Section Rates" *New England Journal of Medicine,* Francis Notzon, et al., 1987, Vol. 316, pgs. 386-389.

"Electronic Fetal Monitoring and Cesarean Section", *New England Journal of Medicine,* correspondence, February 19, 1987;

"Epidurals May Triple C-section Risk" *Medical Tribune for the Obstetrician & Gynecologist,* Susan Ince, February 16, 1995 - Volume 2, Number 4.

"Home Birth After Cesarean" excerpted from *The Home Birth Advantage,* Mayer Eisenstein, M.D., 2000, CMI Press.

"Recent Trends in Cesarean Birth", *JAMA,* Warren Pearse, M.D. et al., 1987; 257:494-497

"Taking Charge of the Cesarean Section Rate" *Family Practice News,* Miriam E. Tucker, January 1, 1997 *Women's Health.*

"The Impact of Cesarean Section in Relation to Fetal Presentation" *American Journal of Obstetrics and Gynecology,* Dr. Rydhstrom, 163:528-533, 1990.

"Trends in the Frequency of Cesarean Births" *Clinical Obstetrics and Gynecology*, Mortimer Rosen, M.D., Vol. 28, No. 4, Dec. 1985

"U.S. Rate of C-sections Stays High" *USA TODAY*, Kim Painter, April 23, 1993

"Vaginal Birth After Cesarean - Controversies Old and New" *Clinical Obstetrics and Gynecology*, Bruce Flamm, M.D., *Clinical Obstetrics and Gynecology*, Vol. 28, No. 4, Dec. 1985

"When Should Labor be Interrupted by Cesarean Delivery?" *Clinical Obstetrics and Gynecology*, Jay Iams, M.D.. Vol. 28, No. 4, Dec. 1985

Chapter III

Unnecessary Birth Interventions

*"None is poor save him
that lacks knowledge"*
Talmud Nedarim

The following scientific studies demonstrate that routine ultrasound, electronic fetal monitoring, induction for PROM (prelabor rupture of membranes), induction for prolonged pregnancy and episiotomy do not increase fetal or maternal well being. These procedures have become standard in obstetrical care and in large part are responsible for the high rate of c-sections (approximately 25% in most hospital practices versus 4% in most home birth practices). Cesarean section is between 2 and 10 times more dangerous for both mother and baby. Our infant and maternal mortality rates, place us last among the top 20 industrial nations. In 1936 Dr. Joseph B. DeLee, considered by many to be the father of modern obstetrics stated. "Yes, there seems to be little doubt that the frequency of cesarean section in our country is one of the causes of our high maternal mortality. Would home delivery, where the temptation to operate is not strong, help the situation any? It seems to in Europe; or should we follow the advise of some and turn the cases back to the midwives?" Sixty four years later we are still struggling with the same problems. For over 70 years doctors have been trying to show, that the hospital is safer than the home for giving birth, only to be amazed, as Dr. DeLee was, that the home produces the better outcome.

It is time for a new obstetrical paradigm. We must look at output measures, not input measures. The newest hospital, newest birthing room, the newest procedures, are all input measures. Output measures would be their cesarean section rate, maternal mortality, infant mortality, etc. In the new paradigm quality in an obstetrical system would be reflected in its cesarean section rate. High cesarean section rate would equal a low quality, a low cesarean rate would equal high quality. As consumers we can have influence on these outcomes. By choosing physicians with low cesarean section rates, we will be avoiding many of the above routine procedures. The best way to accomplish this is by finding physicians and certified nurse midwives who deliver babies at home. The home is the key because the professionals who deliver babies at home believe that "Birth is a normal physiologic process, not a pathological event and operative care should be reserved only where the benefit of the procedure clearly outweighs the risk."

Avoid Electronic Fetal Monitoring

One grossly overused unscientific and dangerous procedure is electronic fetal monitoring. The cover story of *Ob. Gyn. News,* volume 23, number 9, 1988 states that The American College of Obstetricians and Gynecologists' (ACOG) committee on obstetrics has recommended to the ACOG executive board that "periodic auscultation be an acceptable alternative to electronic fetal monitoring for high-risk pregnancies." Auscultation is the listening to fetal heart tones with the use of a head stethoscope on the mother's abdomen.

In the words of Dr. Harold Schulman, a member of the obstetrics committee and Chief of Obstetrics at Winthrop University Hospital, Mineola, NY, "We had come to terms with the accumulating literature showing that fetal monitoring was not only not superior (to auscultation) but may even be dangerous." The article goes on to say that none of eight studies involving nearly 50,000 pregnant women "demonstrated any benefit from electronic fetal monitoring and the results of five indicated that women who were electronically monitored were more likely to undergo cesarean section than those who were not." The maternal mortality rate for cesarean section is 8 to 10 times that of vaginal delivery. Avoiding a cesarean section is the highest priority of the well educated consumer and the science based obstetrical physician.

A 1979 literature review on the efficacy and safety of electronic fetal monitoring co-authored by Banta and Thacker concluded that there was insufficient evidence at that time to recommend the routine use of electronic fetal monitoring. It is ironic that every randomized controlled clinical trial study on electronic fetal monitoring from 1979 through 1996 (see references) shows that electronic fetal monitoring has no scientific validity, yet it is used in virtually every hospital with every laboring woman. Also virtually every scientific study has shown that planned home birth is far safer than planned hospital birth; yet, most doctors won't even consider home birth as an option.

The outstanding individual scientific works from 1973 through 1996 by Drs. Haverkamp, Hon, Landendoerfer, Shy, Nelson, Thacker and Luthy have quite conclusively shown that electronic fetal monitoring is not superior to auscultation. Read the full articles for more detailed information about the futility of electronic fetal monitoring. Please check the list of references.

What has changed with regard to the use of electronic fetal monitoring since 1979? The answer is nothing in the unscientific obstetrical hospital community. Electronic fetal monitoring is still used routinely in spite of the overwhelming scientific evidence that it has no value.

However, the scientific home birth community has virtually abandoned the use of continuous electronic fetal monitoring thereby avoiding the associated risks of increased cesarean section rates. A survey conducted by the American College of Obstetrics and Gynecology shows that the c-section rate is still rising for hospital births.

The home birth philosophy of Homefirst® Health Services comes from Hippocrates the father of modern medicine, "Primum Non Nocere — Above All Do No Harm". Our skilled doctors, certified nurse midwives and nurses, have delivered over 14,000 babies (with hospitalization for cesarean section rate of less than 5%) at home without the use of an electronic fetal monitor. If you are still going to have a baby in the hospital, demand that they will not use continuous electronic fetal monitoring on your baby. Even better, avoid this unnecessary risk altogether, plan to have your baby at home and give you and your baby "The Home Birth Advantage".

Scientific Studies on
Electronic Fetal Monitoring

In the *American Journal Obstetrics Gynecology* 1987; 156:24-30,Stephen B. Thacker, M.D., discussed "The Efficacy of Intrapartum Electronic Fetal Monitoring" and concluded...

"The trials demonstrated no other statistically significant benefit associated with the use of electronic fetal monitoring, but most reported significant increases in the rates of abdominal and vaginal operative deliveries associated with electronic fetal monitoring. Taken together, the seven trials provide valuable information about the routine use of intrapartum electronic fetal monitoring; they do not demonstrate that it is a useful screening procedure for all women in labor."

CBCXCBCX

In the *New England Journal of Medicine* 322:588-593; 1990, Drs. KK Shy, DA Luthy, et al., Univ of Washington; Grace Hosp, Vancouver, studied the "Effects of Electronic Fetal-heart Rate Monitoring, as Compared with Periodic Auscultation On the Neurologic Development of Premature Infants". They concluded that...

"Electronic fetal heart rate monitoring does not lead to improved neurologic development in children born prematurely. It may be less effective than a structured program of periodic auscultation. In this series there was an unanticipated 2.9-fold increase in the odds of having cerebral palsy in the electronically monitored group."

CBCXCBCX

M. H. Klaus, M.D., in the <u>1991 Year Book of Neonatal and Perinatal Medicine</u> comments on the Shy study...

"Though electronic fetal monitoring came in with a flurry with great expectations of reducing central nervous system damage, none of the 8 randomized trials favor its use. I wonder how the routine use of this procedure can be somehow reduced. What amount of data will be required to stop using this procedure routinely?"

M.E. Comments:
As early as 1987 the scientific literature pointed to the conclusion that electronic fetal monitoring did not improve fetal outcome. Why are the results of these studies not implemented?

ଔଔଔଔ

Roger Freeman, M.D., Memorial Medical Center, Long Beach, CA 90801, the author of one of the definitive book on electronic fetal monitoring, commented on the previous major studies on electronic fetal monitoring in an editorial in *The New England Journal of Medicine*, March 1, 1990, 624-626 "Intrapartum Fetal Monitoring - a Disappointing Story" wrote...

"INTRAPARTUM electronic fetal-heart-rate monitoring was introduced in the United States in the early 1970s after studies supported the existence of a correlation between patterns of fetal heart rate and signs of fetal hypoxia—specifically, intrapartum fetal death, fetal blood pH, and Apgar scores. The common perception was that with this objective technique, evidence of fetal hypoxia would appear in a timely fashion, allowing the clinician to intervene and thus protect the fetus from the ravages of continued intrauterine oxygen deprivation....

The first prospective, randomized trial of intrapartum electronic fetal monitoring, by Haverkamp et al., was reported in 1976. It showed no benefit of electronic fetal monitoring as compared with auscultation... There was a higher rate of cesarean birth in the electronic-fetal-monitoring group. A subsequent study of the children involved in the studies of Haverkamp et al. failed to show any long-term benefits of electronic fetal monitoring...

Since then, there have been six prospective, randomized trials of electronic fetal monitoring in a total of 17,510 fetuses born at term. None of these studies found decreases in the rates of intrapartum death, low Apgar scores, or fetal acidosis...

At this point, many loyalists suggested that if there was to be a benefit from electronic fetal monitoring, it would certainly be demonstrated in a randomized trial in premature infants. In 1987 Luthy et al. studied 246 women whose infants weighed between 700 and 1750g, and this study too failed to show any difference in immediate outcome between the infants monitored electronically and those monitored with auscultation.

The article by Shy et al. in this issue of the *Journal* reports a follow-up study of the premature neonates from Luthy's 1987 randomized, controlled trial and examines the outcomes at 18 months with respect to neurologic development. Again, no benefit was found with intrapartum electronic fetal monitoring. The authors point out that the incidence of cerebral palsy among their electronically monitored patients was higher than that reported by others, especially in infants weighing under 1750 g...

Many who had been zealots in the electronic fetal monitoring camp could not explain how a technique that clearly detected fetal hypoxia caused by uteroplacental insufficiency and umbilical cord compression apparently did not lead to beneficial intervention...

Clearly, the hoped-for benefit from intrapartum electronic fetal monitoring has not been realized. It is unfortunate that randomized, controlled trials were not carried out before this form of technology became universally applied. Before we discard the electronic fetal monitor, however, we must realize that the randomized trial all had dedicated nurses assigned to the auscultation group, a circumstance that is not always possible in a busy clinical setting...

The story of electronic fetal monitoring also illustrates the need for proper randomized clinical trials before new forms of technology are introduced that may become the standard of practice without clearly demonstrated benefit."

ଔଔଔଔ

M.E. Comments:

Dr. Freeman, one of the recognized monitoring experts, goes one step short of abandoning electronic fetal monitoring. I find his statement... "Before we discard the electronic fetal monitor, however, we must realize that the randomized trial all had dedicated nurses assigned to the auscultation group, a circumstance that is not always possible in a busy clinical setting". Skilled nurses, certified nurse midwives, and physicians are the makeup of the home birth team. If this is what brings about the healthiest babies and the healthiest mothers let us be straight forward and endorse it. Let us not dance around the issues of the danger of hospital births with its dangerous medical interventions.

ଔଔଔଔ

Michael F. Greene, M.D., Brigham and Women's Hospital, Boston, MA 02115, in his review in the *New England*

Journal of Medicine, of <u>Fetal Heart Rate Monitoring</u>, Second edition by Roger K. Freeman, Thomas J. Garite, and Michael P. Nageotte. 230 pp., illustrated. Baltimore, Williams and Wilkins, 1991 writes...

"Intrapartum electronic monitoring of the fetal heart rate was introduced with great enthusiasm in the early 1970s. It was hoped that with the ability to recognize intrapartum fetal asphyxia and to intervene in a timely fashion, the incidence of neurologic injury to the fetus would be substantially reduced. Specifically, most cases of cerebral palsy were thought to arise during the intrapartum period, and it was hoped that this considerable source of morbidity could essentially be eliminated. Electronic monitoring was quickly adopted, and it became a standard of care by the end of the 1970s. During that decade, hundreds of publications documented associations between various patterns of the fetal heart rate and intrapartum events, medications, and intervention. Residency training programs scheduled weekly monitoring rounds at which "interesting tracings" were intently studied. Barely a whisper of dissent questioning the validity of the technique was heard.

During the 1980s, the utility of the technique was tested in randomized, controlled clinical trials. The first few trials that found no benefit from intrapartum monitoring were criticized for their small size. As such trials grew in size, including one involving almost 35,000 patients that was presented in the *Journal*, and still no benefit was found, they were criticized because they were conducted in term infants at low risk. In 1990 the results of the neurologic evaluations of nearly 200 subjects in a randomized, controlled trial comparing electronic monitoring with intermittent auscultation during labor in premature infants at high risk for intrapartum asphyxia were reported in the *Journal*. This study too found no benefit from monitoring. Commenting in these pages, Roger Freeman characterized intrapartum fetal monitoring as "a disappointing story." In the context of these consistently discouraging results, it might seem incongruous that Freeman and his coauthors are publishing the second edition of his classic work on fetal-heart-rate monitoring. ***Is this monograph a treatise on the pathophysiology of the dodo bird?*** Or is it perhaps (even more harshly) the unicorn? Freeman acknowledges these "disappointments" and notes in his preface that "We are no longer as hopeful that this technology can prevent all or even most cases of cerebral palsy." Nonetheless, electronic monitoring will clearly remain with us for the foreseeable future, if only because it is less expensive than the alternative — skilled nurses.

One hopes that with more modest expectations and
an appreciation of its limited predictive value,
electronic fetal monitoring will serve us better in the
1990s than it has to date."

M.E. Comments:
*Dr. Greene's book review points out that despite the
evidence that EFM produced worse outcomes, change did
not take place. The safety record of physician and certified
nurse midwife home birth attendants, without the use of
unscientific interventions, will be a shining example into the
new millennium for safe childbirth.*

C3C2C3C2

Karin B. Nelson, M.D., et al., in the *New England Journal
of Medicine* 1996; 334:613-8, did a study "Uncertain Value
of Electronic Fetal Monitoring in Predicting Cerebral Palsy"
concluding...

"Electronic monitoring of the fetal heart rate is
commonly performed, in part to detect hypoxia during
delivery that may result in brain injury. It is not
known whether specific abnormalities on electronic
fetal monitoring are related to the risk of cerebral
palsy.

Specific abnormal findings on electronic monitoring
of the fetal heart rate were associated with an
increased risk of cerebral palsy. However, the false

positive rate was extremely high. Since cesarean section is often performed when such abnormalities are noted and is associated with risk to the mother, our findings arouse concern that, if these indications were widely used, many cesarean sections would be performed without benefit and with the potential for harm."

M.E. Comments: Nelson's study in the "New England Journal of Medicine" found that electronic fetal monitoring was commonly performed to detect hypoxia (low oxygen supply to the baby) which could result in brain injury. However, she found that the false positive rate was extremely high. (Many positive findings on the electronic fetal monitor did not result in damaged babies.) This is another in the growing number of studies showing the lack of value in electronic fetal monitoring studies.

ଔଔଔଔ

Jay A. Gold, M.D., J.D., M.P.H. Wisconsin Peer Review Organization Madison, WI 53713, in a letter to the editor in the *New England Journal of Medicine* 1996, 335:287-288, commenting Dr. Nelson's study stated..,.

"Nelson et. al. find that cesarean section is not associated with a significantly altered risk of cerebral palsy in children with multiple late decelerations. Nor, as they point out, was there any evidence that electronic fetal monitoring is associated with improved outcomes. Yet neither the authors nor MacDonald in his editorial comes to the obvious conclusions: that absent special circumstances, electronic fetal monitoring should be abandoned, and that cesarean section (in view of its risks) should not be performed unless there is some indication other than late decelerations.

A greater bluntness would have been desirable. It is difficult enough to bring about a change in physicians' behavior even when a spade is forthrightly called a spade. I fear that many obstetricians who routinely use electronic fetal monitoring and perform cesarean sections for late decelerations will continue to do so as a result of inertia even after they have learned of the study results. I would like to see the authors and the editorialist either endorse the conclusions I draw in no uncertain terms or dispute them."

M.E. Comments:

Gold's commentary on the Nelson study calls for the rightful ending of electronic fetal monitoring.

೮೩೮೩೮೩೮೩

The *Napsac News* Vol. 20, No. 2, Summer 1996, in an article on "Fetal Monitoring" stated...

"In conferences for the general public it is usual to hear an obstetrician demonstrating that electronic fetal monitoring is the most efficient way to detect immediately the beginning of a fetal distress. Nobody can argue with that. It is obvious. The point is that some obstetricians have a major difficulty in understanding that electronic fetal monitoring is, in itself, a *cause* of fetal distress and that the balance between risks and benefits is *negative*. They have not digested the numerous studies demonstrating the negative effects on statistics of an electronic environment. They do not try to understand, for example, why, in a well-known study about premature births, there were 2.5 times more cerebral palsies in the group with electronic fetal monitoring than in the group with intermittent auscultation."

෪ઙ෪ઙ

The U.S. Preventive Task Force Guidelines from Guide to Clinical Preventive Services, (Second Edition) 1996, January 1,1996 Copyright© 1996, Williams & Wilkins, after reviewing the multiple studies on electronic fetal monitoring came to the following conclusions...

"*RECOMMENDATION*

Routine electronic fetal monitoring for low risk women in labor is not recommended. There is insufficient evidence to recommend for or against intrapartum electronic fetal monitoring for high risk pregnant women."

The U.S. Preventive Task Force reviews the recommendation of other groups with regard to electronic fetal monitoring.

"The American College of Obstetrics and Gynecologists states that all patients in labor need some form of fetal monitoring, with more intensified monitoring indicated in high risk pregnancies... The Canadian Task Force on the Periodic Health Examination, advises against routine electronic fetal monitoring in normal pregnancies but found poor evidence regarding the inclusion or exclusion of its routine use in high risk pregnancies."

In discussing these findings they write...

"In addition to the maternal risks associated with electronic fetal monitoring, including increased rates of cesarean or operative vaginal (e.g. forceps) delivery, general anesthesia and maternal infection, and the possible increased risk of adverse neonatal neurologic outcome, increased use of this technology is associated with increased costs of labor care. The widespread use of electronic fetal monitoring in low-risk pregnancies in the face of uncertain benefits, and certain maternal risks and costs, has been attributed to concerns about litigation. It has been estimated that nearly 40% of all obstetric malpractice losses are due to fetal monitoring problems, and this may be a major motivating factor behind the widespread use of electronic fetal monitoring during labor."

The Committee comes to the following conclusion with regard to the clinical intervention of electronic fetal monitoring...

"Routine electronic fetal monitoring is not recommended for low-risk women in labor when adequate clinical monitoring including intermittent auscultation by trained staff is available. There is insufficient evidence to recommend for or against electronic fetal monitoring over intermittent auscultation for high-risk pregnancies. For pregnant women with complicated labor (i.e., induced, prolonged, or oxytocin augmented), recommendations for electronic monitoring plus scalp blood sampling may be made on the basis of evidence for a reduced risk of neonatal seizures, although the long-term neurologic benefit to the neonate is unclear and must be weighed against the increased risk to the mother and neonate of operative delivery, general anesthesia, and maternal infection, and a possible increased risk of adverse neurologic outcome in the infant. There is currently no evidence available to evaluate electronic fetal monitoring in comparison to no monitoring."

M.E. Comments

The above scientific studies on electronic fetal monitoring confirm that routine electronic fetal monitoring has no place in low risk obstetrical care. In fact, the Task Force came to the conclusion that there is not enough evidence to justify any type of monitoring during labor. Maybe nature knew what it was doing with the labor process and our meddlesome obstetrics (high: cesarean section rate; induction rate; ultrasound rate; maternal mortality infant mortality, etc.), have created many of our problems.

REFERENCES FOR ELECTRONIC FETAL MONITORING

Eisenstein M, The Home Birth Advantage, 2000 CMI Press.

Haverkamp A, Orleans M, Langendoerfer S, McFee J, Murphy J, Thompson HE., "A controlled trial of the differential effects of intrapartum fetal monitoring." AM J Obstet Gynecol 1979; 134:399-412.

Haverkamp AD, Thompson HE, McFee JG, Cetrulo C., "The evaluation of continuous fetal heart rate monitoring in high-risk pregnancy." Am J. Obstet Gynecol 1976; 125:310-20.

http://www.homefirst.com

Kelly VC, Kulkarni D., "Experiences with fetal monitoring in a community hospital." Obstet Gynecol 1973: 4:818-24.

Landendoerfer S, Haverkamp AD, Murphy J, et al., "Pediatric follow-up of a randomized controlled trial of intrapartum fetal monitoring techniques." J Pediatr 1980; 97:103-7.

Luthy DA, Shy KK, van Belle G, et al., "A randomized trial of electronic fetal monitoring in preterm labor." Obstet Gynecol 1987; 69:687-95.

Nelson KB, Dambrosia JM, Ting TY, Grether, JK, "Uncertain value of electronic fetal monitoring in predicting cerebral palsy." New England Journal of Medicine 1996; 334:613-8.

Parer JT., "Fetal heart rate monitoring." <u>Lancet</u> 1979; 2:632-3.

Paul RH, Hon EH., "Clinical fetal monitoring. Effect on perinatal outcome." <u>Am J Obstet Gynecol</u> 1974; 188:529-33.

Shy KK, Luth DA, Bennett FC, et al., "Effects of electronic fetal-heart-rate monitoring, as compared with periodic auscultation, on the neurologic development of premature infants." <u>N. Engl J Med</u> 1990; 322:588-93.

Thacker SB, "The efficacy of intrapartum electronic fetal monitoring." <u>Am J Obstet Gynecol</u> 1987; 156:24-30.

Scientifically Unsound
Routine Ultrasound

John P Newnham, et al., in *The Lancet* Vol. 342, October 9, 1993, p. 887-891 reports on "Effects of frequent ultrasound during pregnancy: a randomised controlled study"...

"Despite widespread application of ultrasound imaging and Doppler blood flow studies, the effects of their frequent and repeated use in pregnancy have not been evaluated in controlled trials.... Our findings suggest that five or more ultrasound imaging and Doppler flow studies between 18 and 38 weeks gestation, when compared with a single imaging study at 18 weeks gestation, increases the proportion of growth restricted fetuses by about one third."

ങ്ങരങ്ങ

An editorial in *The Lancet* Vol. 342, October 9, 1993, p. 878. "Frequent prenatal ultrasound: time to think again" comments...

"No medical intervention that offers substantial benefit can ever be entirely harmless. That fact ought to be well known and it applies to ultra sound examination in pregnancy as much as to everything else. Until lately, however, the assumption that ultrasound examination per se was unlikely to have harmful effects was thought reasonable.... The Perth Randomized Controlled Trial of frequent prenatal ultrasound examination [see above reference] brings a cautionary note to that enthusiasm, the message being that prenatal ultrasound by itself can no longer be assumed to be entirely harmless.... There are several well documented benefits of Doppler flow measurements in high risk pregnancy. This fact does not necessarily mean that prenatal ultrasound is a harmless intervention. Clearly it is prudent to limit such examinations to circumstances in which the information is likely to be useful."

03CR03CR

Ewigman, Bernard, et al, *New England Journal of Medicine*, September 16, 1993, Vol 329, pp 821-827, discusses the conclusions from his randomized controlled trial in"Effects of Prenatal Ultrasound Screening on Perinatal Outcome"...

"Many clinicians advocate routine ultrasound screening during pregnancy to detect congenital anomalies, multiple-gestation pregnancies, fetal growth disorders, placental abnormalities, and errors in the estimation of gestational age. However, it is not known whether the detection of these conditions through screening leads to interventions that improve perinatal outcome.

We conducted a randomized trial involving 15,151 pregnant women at low risk for perinatal problems to determine whether ultrasound screening decreased the frequency of adverse perinatal outcomes. The women randomly assigned to the ultrasound-screening group underwent one sonographic examination at 15 to 22 weeks of gestation and another at 31 to 35 weeks. The women in the control group underwent ultrasonography only for medical indications, as identified by their physicians. Adverse perinatal outcome was defined as fetal death, neonatal death, or neonatal morbidity such as intra ventricular hemorrhage.

The mean numbers of sonograms obtained per woman in the ultrasound-screening and control groups were 2.2 and 0.6, respectively. The rate of adverse perinatal outcome was 5.0 percent among the infants of the women in the ultrasound-screening group and 4.9 percent among the infants of the women in the control group.... The rates of preterm delivery and the distribution of birth weights were nearly identical in the two groups. The ultrasonographic detection of congenital anomalies had no effect on perinatal outcome. There were no significant differences between the groups in perinatal outcome in the subgroups of women with post-date pregnancies, multiple-gestation pregnancies, or infants who were small for gestational age.

Screening ultrasonography did not improve perinatal outcome as compared with the selective use of ultrasonography on the basis of clinician judgment."

ඔඔඔඔ

The U.S. Preventive Task Force <u>Guidelines from Guide to Clinical Preventive Services</u>, (Second Edition) 1996, January 1,1996 Copyright © 1996, Williams & Wilkins, after reviewing the multiple studies on *Screening Ultrasonography in Pregnancy* came to the following conclusions:

"RECOMMENDATION
Routine third-trimester ultrasound examination of the fetus is not recommended. There is insufficient evidence to recommend for or against routine ultrasound examination in the second trimester in low-risk pregnant women."

In discussing these findings they write...
"Neither early, late, nor serial ultrasound in normal pregnancy has been proven to improve perinatal morbidity or mortality. Clinical trials show that a single mid-trimester ultrasound examination detects

multiple gestations and congenital malformations earlier in pregnancy, but there is currently insufficient evidence that early detection results in improved outcomes."

The Committee comes to the following conclusion with regard to the clinical intervention of routine ultra sound examination...

"Routine ultrasound examination of the fetus in the third trimester is not recommended, based on multiple trials and meta-analyses showing no benefit for either the pregnant woman or her fetus. There is currently insufficient evidence to recommend for or against a single routine mid-trimester ultrasound in low-risk pregnant women. These recommendations apply to routine screening ultrasonography and not to diagnostic ultrasonography for specific clinical indications."

M.E. COMMENTS:

Obstetrical ultrasound, just like electronic fetal monitoring has become a standard of hospital based obstetrical care without any scientific evidence that ultrasound provides better maternal and/or fetal outcomes. Because doctors' beliefs trump scientific evidence, we continue to be exposed to dangerous and costly procedures. Obstetrical ultrasound has been heralded as a 100% safe medical procedure.

However, as Newnham, et al., point out in the "Lancet" study, multiple exposure to ultrasound correlates with growth restriction in fetuses. The accompanying editorial superbly states "No medical intervention that offers substantial benefit can ever be entirely harmless." That statement sums it all up. We must weigh with any medical procedure the risk versus the benefit. Only when the benefits outweigh the risks, should we recommend a particular medical procedure. Maybe the scientific evidence will eventually show that for routine ultrasound the benefits will outweigh the risks. However, as we have learned from electronic fetal monitoring, vaccines, antibiotics, etc. nothing is 100% risk free.

REFERENCES FOR ULTRA SOUND

Editorial, "Frequent prenatal ultrasound: time to think again". The Lancet Vol. 342, October 9, 1993, p. 878.

Ewigman, Bernard, et al,"Effects of Prenatal Ultrasound Screening on Perinatal Outcome." New England Journal of Medicine, September 16, 1993, Vol 329, pp 821-827.

John P Newnham, et al.,"Effects of frequent ultrasound during pregnancy: a randomised controlled study". The Lancet Vol. 342, October 9, 1993, p. 887-891.

U.S. Preventive Task Force "Screening Ultrasonography in Pregnancy". Guidelines from Guide to Clinical Preventive Services, (Second Edition) 1996, January 1,1996 Copyright © 1996, Williams & Wilkins.

Scientifically Unsound
Routine Induction
of Labor for Prolonged Pregnancy

In the *International Journal of Gynaecological Obstetrics* pp. 145-147, 1995, Ohel G; Yaacobi N, et al, studied "Postdate Antenatal Testing" and concluded...

"Perinatal morbidity and mortality is increased with postmaturity. For each week of gestation after 40 weeks, the complications increase significantly. Fetal testing typically begins at 42 weeks, but recent reports indicate earlier testing may be warranted. The impact of very early postdate testing, which was begun within a few days of confinement, was studied.

...Early fetal surveillance beginning at 40 weeks still resulted in a higher incidence of emergency cesarean sections, meconium in the amniotic fluid, and heavy infants in postdate pregnancies."

T.H. Kirschbaum, M.D., Professor, Department of Obstetrics and Gynecology, Albert Einstein College of Medicine, commenting in the Year Book of Obstetrics and Gynecology® 1996, Copyright © 1996 Mosby-Year Book, Inc. Vol. 49 on the Ohel, et al, study wrote...

"Although it seems that the incidence of obstetric and neonatal problems increases in pregnancies past (280 days of gestation, it does not necessarily follow that surveillance of those fetuses at and past that point in gestation suffices to abolish those problems.... The surveillance regimen [in the above study] was unable to prevent an increasing incidence of cesarean section, fetal distress, uterine dysfunction, meconium staining, and macrosomia past 40 weeks. The authors' conclusions suggest that, although it is of no particular advantage for a fetus to be born post dates, existing management protocols don't enable us to prevent the association with obstetric problems."

ෲ෬ෲ෬

In the *British Journal of Obstetrics and Gynaecology,* 105:169-173, 1998, Hilder L, et al., studied "Prolonged Pregnancy: Evaluating Gestation-specific Risks of Fetal and Infant Mortality" and concluded...

"The risks of prolonged pregnancy include meconium aspiration, birth injury, and hypoxia, and fetal loss...

No significant differences were seen between stillbirth rates at term and post-term...

A more accurate method of determining the risks of prolonged gestation on pregnancy is by calculating fetal and infant loss per 1,000 ongoing pregnancies. In prolonged pregnancy, the risk of stillbirth and neonatal and postneonatal mortality are significantly higher. These data may help pregnant women and health care providers make decisions about obstetric intervention."

T.H. Kirschbaum, M.D., Professor, Department of Obstetrics and Gynecology, Albert Einstein College of Medicine, commenting in the Year Book of Obstetrics, Gynecology, and Women's Health@ 1999, pages 41-42, Copyright © 1999 Mosby, Inc., on the Hilder L, et al., study wrote...

"Whether perinatal mortality is increased after either 41 or 42 completed weeks of gestation remains controversial in our literature, and this study of births registered from 18 regional hospitals in London helps explain some of the confusion.... Remember that attempts to improve the survival in postdates pregnancy, regardless of the estimated risks, has never been demonstrated uniformly. This experience helps support the contention that the risk of stillborn is not increased in postdate pregnancy."

ଔଔଔଔ

In the *American Journal of Obstetrics and Gynecology* 70:716—723. 1994, Mosby, Inc., McNellis D. did a study, "A Clinical Trial of Induction of Labor Versus Expectant Management in Postterm Pregnancy" and concluded...

"In uncomplicated pregnancies that pass the estimated date of birth, the benefits of reducing the potential fetal risk with induction of labor must be weighed against the morbidity associated with inducing labor. Two strategies for managing post-term pregnancy—immediate induction and expectant management—were compared.

...The incidence of adverse perinatal outcomes, such as neonatal seizures, intra cranial hemorrhage, the need for mechanical ventilation, or nerve injury, was 1.5% in the induction group and 1% in the expectant management group.

...Adverse perinatal outcomes are rare in uncomplicated pregnancies of 41 weeks or more that are treated by either induction or expectant management schemes. Therefore, either scheme is acceptable."

T.H. Kirschbaum, M.D., Professor, Department of Obstetrics and Gynecology, Albert Einstein College of Medicine, in the **Year Book of Obstetrics, Gynecology, and**

Women's Health@ 1995, pages 75,76, Copyright © 1995 commenting on the McNellis study wrote...

>...What can be concluded is that the bulk of morbidity associated with postdatism rests in the incidental medical and obstetric complications of postdatism, and that management that is based upon this conclusion, when modified by estimates of amniotic fluid volume and the use of the NST (also of unproven efficacy), settles management decisions in most cases. For the rest of the patients who met these entry criteria but who failed to express those concerns in question, it did not seem to matter how long they remained pregnant."

෫ൟ෫ൟ

M.E. Comments:

Here is another way to lower cesarean section rates. Avoid hospital based doctors who routinely induce women for prolonged pregnancy.

**REFERENCES FOR ROUTINE INDUCTION
OF LABOR FOR PROLONGED PREGNANCY**

Editorial, Kirschbaum, T.H., M.D. <u>Year Book of Obstetrics, Gynecology, and Women's Health@ 1999</u>, Copyright © 1999 Mosby, Inc., pages 41,42.

Editorial, Kirschbaum, T.H., M.D., <u>Year Book of Obstetrics and Gynecology</u>® 1996, Copyright © 1996 Mosby-Year Book, Inc. Vol. 49.

Editorial, Kirschbaum, T. H., M.D., <u>Year Book of Obstetrics, Gynecology, and Women's Health@ 1995</u>, Copyright © 1995 Mosby, Inc., pages 73,74.

Hilder L, et al., "Prolonged Pregnancy: Evaluating Gestation-specific Risks of Fetal and Infant Mortality" <u>British Journal of Obstetrics and Gynaecology</u>, 105:169-173, 1998.

McNellis D., "A Clinical Trial of Induction of Labor Versus Expectant Management in Postterm Pregnancy", <u>American Journal of Obstetrics and Gynecology</u> 70:716-723,1994.

Ohel G; Yaacobi N, et al, "Postdate Antenatal Testing" the <u>International Journal of Gynaecological Obstetrics</u> pp. 145-147, 1995.

Scientifically Unsound; Routine Use of Induction for Prelabor Rupture of Membranes

In the *Journal of Perinatal Medicine* - 1996; 24(6): 563-72, Keirse MJ et al. studied "Controversies: prelabor rupture of the membranes at term: the case for expectant management" and concluded...

"Review of the controlled comparisons between induction of labor and expectant care after prelabor rupture of the membranes (PROM) at term indicates that they are not unhelpful for deciding which of the two options is best. This is, first, because there is a large potential for bias in the studies reported thus far. Second, the trials are rather heterogeneous and they are comparisons more between early and late induction than between induction and expectant care. Third, it is difficult to weigh an increased risk of operative delivery with the induction policy against an apparently clear, but almost certainly biased, reduction of neonatal infection. With expectant care about 70% of women will give birth within 24 hours and 85% within 48 hours. **The majority of these women will derive little, if any, benefit from induction and a routine policy of induction of labor**

after PROM cannot be justified on the basis of the data that are available."

෪෬෪෬

In the *New England Journal of Medicine* 1996;334: 1005-10 Mary E. Hannah, et al., studied Prelabor Rupture Of Membranes at Term and concluded...

"As the interval between rupture of the fetal membranes at term and delivery increases, so may the risk of fetal and maternal infection. It is not known whether inducing labor will reduce this risk or whether one method of induction is better than another...

The rates of neonatal infection and cesarean section were not significantly different among the study groups...

In women with prelabor rupture of the membranes at term, induction of labor with oxytocin or prostaglandin E($_2$) and expectant management result in similar rates of neonatal infection and cesarean section..."

෪෬෪෬

M.E. Comments:

You just wonder why, with no scientific justification for routine induction for prelabor rupture of membranes, why has this intervention become the standard of obstetrical care? "I think therefore I believe" are the operative words. Home birth physicians have historically abandoned routine induction of labor for PROM. They are true scientists.

REFERENCES

Hannah, Mary E., et al., "Prelabor Rupture Of Membranes at Term". New England Journal of Medicine 1996;334: 1005-10,

Keirse MJ, et al., "Controversies: prelabor rupture of the membranes at term: the case for expectant management". Journal of Perinatal Medicine 1996; 24(6): 563-72.

Scientific Studies on
Routine Episiotomy

In the *Obstetrical and Gynecologic* Survey 1983, June; 38(6): 322-38, Stephen B. Thacker, M.D., discussed "Benefits and Risks of Episiotomy: An Interpretive Review of the English Language Literature, 1860 Through 1980," and concluded...

"The benefits and risks of episiotomy in labor and delivery as recorded in the English language literature in over 350 books and articles published since 1860 are reviewed and analyzed. Episiotomy is performed in over 60 per cent of all deliveries in the United States and in a much higher per cent of primigravidas (first time mothers). Yet, there is no clearly defined evidence for its efficacy, particularly for routine use. In addition, although poorly studied, there is evidence that postpartum pain and discomfort are accentuated after episiotomy, and serious complications, including maternal death, can be associated with the procedure. Therefore, carefully designed controlled trials of benefit and risk should be carried out on the use of episiotomy."

છા ૨છા ૨

In *Lancet* 1993; 342: 1517-18, Dr. Belizan discussed, "Routine vs. Selective Episiotomy: A Randomized Controlled Trial" and concluded...

"Episiotomy is a widely-done intervention in childbirth, regardless of poor scientific evidence of its benefits... Anterior perineal trauma was more common in the selective group but posterior perineal surgical repair, perineal pain, healing complications, and dehiscence were all less frequent in the selective group. **Routine episiotomy should be abandoned and episiotomy rates above 30% cannot be justified...** There is, then, no reliable evidence that routine use of episiotomy has any beneficial effect, and there is clear evidence that it may cause harm.

Cଃଓଃଓଃଓଃ

In the *Canadian Medical Association Journal*, 1995, Sep. 15; 153(g): 783-6, Dr. M.C. Klein, et al., studied "Physicians' beliefs and behaviour during a randomized controlled trial of episiotomy: consequences for women in their care" and concluded...

"Physicians with favourably views of episiotomy were more likely to use techniques to expedite labour, and their patients were more likely to have perineal trauma and to be less satisfied with the birth experience. This evidence that physician beliefs can influence patient outcomes has both clinical and research implications."

M.E. Comments:

Another example of "I think, therefore I believe."

CRCRCRCR

In the *American Journal of Obstetrics and Gynecology* 1997 Feb;176(2):498-9, Lede, RL, et al., studied "Is routine use of episiotomy justified?" and concluded...

"Episiotomy, one of the most common surgical procedures, was introduced in clinical practice in the eighteenth century without having strong scientific evidence of its benefits... In relation to long-term effects, women in whom management includes routine use of episiotomy have shown poorer future sexual function, similar pelvic floor muscle strength, and similar urinary incontinence in comparison with women in whom episiotomy is used in a selective manner... In view of the available evidence the routine use of episiotomy should be abandoned and episiotomy rates> 30% do not seem justified.

CRCRCRCR

In *Obstetrics and Gynecology Clinics of North America,* 1999 Jun; 26(2): *305-25,* Myers-Helfgott, MG, et al., studied "Routine use of episiotomy in modern obstetrics. Should it be performed?" and concluded...

"Episiotomy... has been associated with a more difficult and lengthy repair as measured by the need for suture material and operating room time. The claims of a protective effect on the fetus in shortening the second stage of labor, improving Apgar scores, and preventing perinatal asphyxia have not been borne out. The value of episiotomy use on a routine basis bears scientific examination in prospective, randomized, controlled trials. These types of trials are certainly achievable, ethically correct, and much needed. Until these trials are completed and published, obstetricians should not routinely perform the procedure but rather determine the need for episiotomy on a case-by-case basis.

ᘓᘂᘓᘂ

In the *Wall Street Journal*, Vol. CV, No. 64, March 30, 2000, Section A, page 1, Chase, Marilyn, reported on, "A Commonly Used Aid To Childbirth Faces Doubts About Benefits — Episiotomy, Once Routine, May Not Ease Delivery And Can Slow Recovery"...

"Once considered the kindest cut, episiotomy has been performed on millions of American women for its supposed benefits; surprisingly, statistics suggest it wasn't such a good deal. Tomorrow, yet another medical research paper [*The British Medical Journal*] makes the argument that the procedure has been overused. Across the U.S., a number of hospitals have begun pulling back from the procedure, dramatically reducing the number of episiotomies they perform... The reign of tradition over data so irked famed British epidemiologist Archie Cochrane that he awarded a wooden spoon - the British equivalent of a booby prize - to obstetrics for being the least scientific of all medical specialties... One of its key findings, in a 1995 review and again last year [1999], is that routine episiotomy adds to the trauma, suturing and complications of delivery...

And what do women want in 2000? 'They've read well enough to know they want a non-interventionist delivery'".

ଓଷଓଷଓଷଓଷ

M.E. Comments

It seems that Ms. Chase from the "Wall Street Journal" has got it right. Women want non-interventionists for delivery. That is exactly what home birth physicians and home birth certified nurse midwives are all about. The scare tactics of hospital based doctors has led to the very shameful results of high cesarean section rate, high infant mortality, and high maternal mortality. Let us hope and pray that the scientific approach to obstetrics will prevail in the 21st century and that non-interventionist home birth doctors and home birth midwives will be the providers of this scientific standard of care.

REFERENCES

Belizan, Dr., "Routine vs. Selective Episiotomy: A Randomized Controlled Trial." Lancet 1993; 342: 1517-18.

Chase, Marilyn, "A Commonly Used Aid To Childbirth Faces Doubts About Benefits — Episiotomy, Once Routine, May Not Ease Delivery And Can Slow Recovery" *Wall Street Journal*, Vol. CV, No. 64, March 30, 2000, Section A, page 1.

Klein, M.C. Dr., et al., "Physicians' beliefs and behaviour during a randomized controlled trial of episiotomy: consequences for women in their care" Canadian Medical Association Journal, 1995, Sep. 15; 153(g): 783-6.

Lede, RL, et al., "Is routine use of episiotomy justified?" American Journal of Obstetrics and Gynecology 1997 Feb;176(2):498-9,

Myers-Helfgott, MG, et al., "Routine use of episiotomy in modern obstetrics. Should it be performed?" Obstetrics and Gynecology Clinics of North America, 1999 Jun; 26(2): 305-25.

Thacker, Stephen B. M.D., "Benefits and Risks of Episiotomy: An Interpretive Review of the English Language Literature, 1860 Through 1980" Obstetrical and Gynecologic Survey 1983, June; 38(6): 322-38.

Chapter IV

Breastfeeding

"Breasts are more skillful at compounding a feeding mixture than the hemispheres of the most learned professor's brain."

- Oliver Wendel Holmes, M.D.

Information And Support Are Essential To Success

A *Family Health Forum* listener related a personal story to my radio audience. When she was a new mother, she was determined to nurse her daughter. "Nursing just had to work for me," she said on the air, "because everything else about her hospital delivery was so disappointing. We had planned for a natural delivery but in the hospital had one unnecessary intervention after another. The natural experience of nursing became very important to me after our unnatural birth experience."

"My doctor told me to wash my breasts with sterile water before and after each feeding. In no time this advice created a disaster. I developed a terrible rash on both breasts. I was very uncomfortable and nursing was quite painful. My breasts were cracked, bleeding and itchy. When I could no longer stand it, I sought the advice of another doctor who told me to stop washing my breasts. I had developed eczema from the constant irritation of the sterile water." The listener shared her unfortunate story to show the disastrous effects of incorrect nursing information. "Even though I am a doctor, my breastfeeding knowledge was limited to a few lectures in medical school. Doctors just don't learn much about it. So I didn't know that there is no need for special washing before or after nursing."

"All women should go to La Leche League even before their babies are born," she recommends. "This will increase tremendously their ability to nurse and to enjoy nursing their babies. Doctors are complicating and even terminating nursing for many mothers and babies based on doctor myths about breastfeeding. There is no better source of support and information than La Leche League."

Nursing Means Superior Health

I only semi-jokingly have said that this chapter should be one sentence long. Our one sentence chapter would read, "Do it!"

In some ways breastfeeding a baby is as simple a concept as home birth. It gives infants the best start in life and maintains optimum health.

I was taught in medical school that breast and bottle feeding were about the same. But during the years I have been in practice, study after study has consistently shown that nutritionally, psychologically, and medically, nursing is superior to bottle feeding.

In our practice (Homefirst® Health Services) we see virtually 100% nursing infants. Over the years we have cared for over 30,000 children, with very few cases of allergies, eczema, asthma, ear infections, bronchitis, pneumonia, etc.. Nursing dramatically improves the health of infants, decreasing the probability of them having these problems.

You Can't Fool Mother Nature!

We will continue to promote nursing because it is right. Mother nature is the supreme healer and provider of superior nutrition for infants. There will never be a formula that can substitute for mother's milk. There will never be a relationship so important to our children's health as the mother/child nursing relationship.

Nursing is a very natural and instinctive process all mothers are capable of doing successfully if the medical professional establishment does not interfere. This was explained so well in an address by Dr. Herbert Ratner on "The Natural Institution of the Family", in 1987. He said to the tenth convention of the Fellowship of Catholic Scholars, "Jesus, for instance, tells us to love our neighbor. But Jesus does not instruct the mother how to love her closest and dearest neighbor, the newborn. Thus the mother is not told to nurse or breastfeed her baby. [Jesus] assumes that with eyes to see, with the milk dripping from postpartum breasts, with hungry suckling lips rooting in search of the mother's teats, the woman can figure this out for herself."

Breastfeeding

No matter how much knowledge a mother has, no matter how much education, the mother who accepts nature, not the doctor, as possessing wisdom, need not know the reason but she remains ahead of science.

Artificial feeding is an attempt to fool nature but the bottom line is that it can't happen. Our society is paying heavily with the health and very lives of our children by providing an inferior imitation of nature's nutritional plan. Breast milk is a precious natural resource that we, in our society, are all too willing to waste. It is every bit as essential to our children's growth as adequate rainfall is to the growth of our farmers' crops.

The late Dr. Robert Mendelsohn said that it is imperative for physicians to demand that mothers nurse. Bottle feeding places the health and welfare of infants in our society at risk. There is certainly truth in his words. Every year in the United States there are three million infants born. They are born into a society which doesn't promote nursing and many of them die of complications from the inferior substitutes they are fed. The United States has the highest infant mortality rate among the top twenty industrialized nations. The use of infant formula has helped to place us in the last position and will help to keep us there if its use continues.

Scientists have been trying for over fifty years to reproduce breast milk and they have not been successful. Every mother produces milk unique to her baby and its needs. It has been discovered that mothers of premature infants produce milk higher in caloric content that than produced for full-term infants. It is nature's way of helping the very small infants gain weight faster, thereby attempting to make up for their prematurity.

The great doctor Oliver Wendel Holmes once said, "Breasts are more skillful at compounding a feeding mixture than the hemispheres of the most learned professor's brain." This has certainly proven to be true. Over 100 different components in breast milk have been isolated so far, with an additional one or two being discovered each year.

Formula is no magic concoction. Anyone who reads the ingredients on a can of infant formula will see that it is simply a recipe of cow's milk, sugar and water. While cow's milk is nature's perfect milk for calves, human milk is nature's perfect milk for humans.

 C3C2C3C3

In the *New England Journal of Medicine* - July 30, 1992, Jukka Karjalainen, M.D., et al., studied *Critical Scientific Analysis of* "A BOVINE ALBUMIN PEPTIDE (cow's milk protein as found in infant formula as well as all forms of milk) AS A POSSIBLE TRIGGER OF INSULIN-DEPENDENT JUVENILE DIABETES MELLITUS"

Mark Zumhagen, M.D. an Attending Physician with Homefirst® Health Services and a Board Certified Diplomate

Breastfeeding

of the American Board of Quality Assurance and Utilization Review Physicians reviewed the Karjalainen study and concluded...

"This scholarly, scientific research has been conducted over a 10-15 year period, it is not just something that has been stumbled upon. It is the result of some very careful scientific scrutiny and detective work to really come up with this connection between the use of cow's milk in the first year of life and the subsequent development of juvenile onset diabetes mellitus.

The researchers were able to isolate one particular protein (out of several hundred) in cow's milk that was responsible for this problem. With this particular protein, there seems to be a correlation with antibodies being developed against this protein and the subsequent development of juvenile diabetes in certain susceptible young patients.

They discovered that this particular protein consists of over 800 amino acids, 17 of which are really responsible for the problem. The researchers were able to identify the small spot on the protein that causes the problem. The way the problem develops is the particular sequence of amino acids very much parallels a similar strand of amino acids that exist in the human pancreas on the beta cells of the pancreas. When the body builds up an antibody against this foreign cow's milk protein, the antibodies are in a sense fooled; they don't recognize the difference between the cow's milk protein and the beta pancreas cell protein, because there is this similar chain of amino acids. Once you have the antibody against the cow's milk protein, you also have an antibody that is going to attack the pancreas cell. Once the pancreas cells have been destroyed the person becomes a diabetic, as they are unable to produce insulin.

The three most commonly asked questions that I tried to address were:

Q) Does this mean that every child that is on formula (the main ingredient of formula is cow's milk which contains this bovine albumin peptide) in the first year of life is going to develop diabetes?

A) The answer is no. Juvenile diabetes develops only in a small percentage of children that are predisposed to develop these antibodies through the cross reaction. So, while there is always a risk that it can happen, it does not happen in the majority of babies that are fed formula.

Q) If the child starts drinking milk after one year of age, will this cross reaction still occur, resulting in juvenile diabetes?

A) The answer again is no because, as the child matures (over one year of age), it no longer absorbs large segments of protein. The proteins are broken down to such a degree that this string of 17 amino acids no longer exists for the antibodies to be formed against.

Q) Why does diabetes develop when the child is anywhere from 5 to 25 years old, if this occurred during the first year of life?
A) The answer is because the pancreatic cells (the beta cells which produce insulin) aren't destroyed in a rapid fashion. The body thinks that the section of the beta cell that resembles this string of 17 amino acids, is a foreign protein on the pancreas and thus it destroys it. In fact this beta cell is only brought to the surface of the pancreas during episodes of illness. Only after a period of time, after whatever illnesses the child goes through in the first few years of life, does the complete destruction of the beta cells occur, rendering the child unable to produce insulin, and thus becoming diabetic.

But the major point is that it is amazing that it has taken us more than 50 years of having a large percentage of our population bottlefeed to discover this link and it is a link that nobody really could have predicted. It seems like such an unlikely thing to happen, but it points out the susceptibility of children under a year of age to any type of foreign substance utilization. Any type of foreign protein or substance (i.e. medication, infant formula made from cow's milk or soy, etc.) introduced into their bodies, has to be done with extreme caution, because this is a time, the first 9-12 months of life, when major problems can occur because the infant's body is still in the process of maturation.

It has taken over 50 years to discover the connection between infant formula (cow's milk) and juvenile diabetes and this points out the need to be very careful and cautious about any type of foreign substance introduced in the child's first year of life. This is just one more bit of evidence to demonstrate the extreme superiority of breastfeeding. As a physician, this leaves us with no choice but to singularly recommend breastfeeding."

ೞೞೞೞ

Financial Savings to Government and Families by Breastfeeding

A pre-publication study by the Wisconsin State Breastfeeding Coalition estimated the following health care savings in Wisconsin if breastfeeding rates were at 75% at discharge-50% at six months:

Breastfeeding

- $4,645,250/yr Acute Otitis Media
- $437,120/yr Bronchitis
- $6,699,600/yr Gastroenteritis
- $262,440/yr Allergies
- $758,934/yr Asthma
- $578,500/yr Type I Diabetes (birth-18 yrs)
- 17,070,000/yr Breast Cancer
- **$30,984,432/yr TOTAL HEALTH COST SAVINGS**

M.E. Comments:

*The 31 million dollar total health cost savings from breastfeeding would translate into **1.5 BILLION** dollars in health cost savings for the entire United States of America. The health benefits of breastfeeding can now actually be calculated into dollars and cents. We do have a health care crisis in this country and breastfeeding is one way to solve a major part of it.*

ଔଔଔଔ

Shortly before James P. Grant, Executive Director of UNICEF, passed away in 1994 he wrote this letter asking support from physicians world wide.

Call to Physicians for Support

Dear Physician,

I smoked cigarettes for years. Then evidence about smoking's ill effects began to mount and finally, no longer able to ignore medical advice, I decided to stop. Like me, many other former smokers are indebted to their physicians. Doctors led the public to appreciate the dangers of smoking. The scientific community has now recognized a parallel threat to our children. I am writing to ask for your help and leadership in disarming it.

Physicians have long known that "breast is best," but there is now increasing awareness that breastfeeding plays a far more crucial role in the survival and healthy development of children—in industrialized and developing countries alike—than we ever before imagined. Study after study now shows, for example, that babies who are not breastfed have higher rates of death, meningitis, childhood leukemia and other cancers, diabetes, respiratory illnesses, bacterial and viral infections, diarrhoea diseases, otitis media, allergies, obesity and developmental delays. Women who do not breastfed demonstrate a higher risk for breast and ovarian cancers.

Despite these facts, too few health care providers inform their patients about a mother's extraordinary capacity to sustain and protect human life— her children's and her own. Even the manufacturers agree that no formula can provide the immunological factors found in human milk. Breastmilk's complex mixture of micro nutrients is unequaled for optimal physical and neurological development. Because products used as substitutes for breastmilk are definitely inferior to it and contribute to increased rates of illness, they cannot legitimately be described as health products. Their marketing has no place in our health systems.

Incredibly, however, substantial quantities of free infant formula are still routinely distributed through hospitals and doctors' offices in the 1990's. Manufacturers regularly provide free and low-cost bulk supplies and individual samples to hospitals, clinics and other parts of the health care system, and well-meaning doctors and nurses then complete the marketing plan by passing the products along to patients, or by providing coupons for free supplies. When substitutes for breastmilk are distributed in health care settings by physicians and other trusted health professionals, the implication is that these products are the better more modern and doctor recommended feeding choice.

I am writing to ask you to take the lead in bringing about the necessary reform of this harmful, outdated habit. It will take the commitment of forward-thinking physicians to let others know that such marketing not only discourages breastfeeding, but also gives mothers the false impression that there are equally healthy alternatives. The weight of your influence, reputation and example can help end unhealthy competition against breast- feeding—competition that is nowhere less appropriate than within our health care systems.

In May, the Member States of the United Nations sent their public health professionals to the World Health Assembly to speak in one voice. By global consensus, they urged all countries to close this dangerous chapter in the history of health care—to end the distribution of free and low-cost supplies of breastmilk substitutes throughout the world's health care systems. Perhaps your voice was among those calling for an end to this dangerously misleading practice. If you did not have the opportunity to speak for your government at the World Health Organization, I urge you now to join an international vanguard of physicians by sending the United Nations your personal pledge to protect breastfeeding. A 'Physician's Pledge' form is printed overleaf for your signature.

Our first goal has been to draw media attention to this crucial child health issue during World Breastfeeding Week, 1-7 August. I am hoping that, with your pledge and the pledges of other concerned physicians in hand, the public will hear that a change of direction is urgently needed and that prominent physicians have stepped forward to lead the way.

Will you take a stand with UNICEF to protect breastfeeding? I look forward to receiving your signed pledge during World Breastfeeding Week, or during the upcoming weeks as our vanguard continues to grow.

Yours sincerely,

James P. Grant

CXCXCXCX

PHYSICIAN'S PLEDGE TO PROTECT, PROMOTE AND SUPPORT BREASTFEEDING

RECOGNIZING that breastfeeding plays a uniquely important role in the healthy development of infants and young children:

...that no substitute can provide the complex balance of nutrients, antibodies and growth factors that make breastmilk the perfect food for infants;

...that women have the right to make infant feeding decisions based on complete and accurate information;

...that my role as a physician is one of influence, authority and trust;

...that breastfeeding is an endangered natural resource that requires my protection, promotion and support;

...the current marketing practices — including the free and low-cost distribution of breastmilk substitute supplies

to hospitals and other parts of the health care system —
compete against and discourage breastfeeding;

...that my Government, at the 1994 World Health
Assembly, affirmed that the marketing and promotion of
breastmilk substitutes should not be conducted anywhere in
the health care system; and

...that the promotion of health and the prevention of
disease are my duties and the mandates of responsible
health care providers everywhere.

ଓଷଔଷଓଷଔଷ

World Health Organization/UNICEF Joint Statement
Every facility providing maternity services and care for
newborn infants should:

1) Have a written breastfeeding policy which is routinely
communicated to all healthcare staff.

2) Train all healthcare staff in skills necessary to
implement this policy.

3) Inform all pregnant women about the benefits and
management of breastfeeding.

4) Help mothers initiate breastfeeding within ½ hour of
birth.

5) Show mothers how to breastfed and how to maintain
lactation even if they should be separated from their infants.

6) Give newborn infants no food or drink other than
breast milk unless medically indicated.

Breastfeeding

7) Practice rooming in - allow mothers and infants to remain together 24 hours a day.

8) Encourage breastfeeding on demand.

9) Give no artificial teats or pacifiers (also called dummies or soothers) to breastfeeding infants.

10) Foster the establishment of breastfeeding support groups and refer mothers to them upon discharge from the hospital or clinic.

M.E. Comments: *Ask your physician if he/she is willing to take the UNICEF Pledge to protect, promote and support breastfeeding. Since there are no safe alternative to breastfeeding, if your physician is not willing to accept this pledge, I recommend that you find another physician.*

ෆ෪ෆ෪

REFERENCES

(The following is a small sampling from over 1,000 scientific articles which demonstrate the serious health and economic hazards of cow's milk labeled as formula.)

Increased Infections

Diarrhea

Children less than 12 months of age had a lower incidence of acute diarrheal disease during the months they were being breastfed than children that were fed with formula during the same period. Lerman, Y. et al. "Epidemiology of acute diarrheal diseases in children in a high standard of living settlement in Israel".

Pediatric Infectious Disease Journal 1994; 13(2); 116-22

Ear Infection

Significantly increased risk for acute otitis media as well as prolonged duration of middle ear effusion were associated with male gender, sibling history of ear infection and not being breastfed. Teele, D.W.,"Epidemiology of Otitis Media During the First Seven Years of Life in Greater Boston: A Prospective Cohort Study".   *Journal of Infectious Diseases, 1989*

Respiratory Viral Infections (RSV)

Breastfeeding was associated with a lower incidence of RSV infection during the first year of life. Holberg, C. J.,

"Risk Factors for RSV Associated Lower Respiratory Illnesses in the First Year of Life".

American Journal Epidemiology, 1991; 133 (135-51)

Increased Incidence of Diseases

Wheezing

Breastfeeding seems to protect against wheezing, respiratory tract illnesses in the first 4 months of life, particularly when other risk factors are present. Wright, A.L., "Breastfeeding and Lower Respiratory Tract Illnesses in the First Year of Life".

British Medical Journal, 1989

Sudden Infant Death Syndrome (SIDS)

Not breastfeeding at discharge from an obstetric hospital at any stage of the infant's life was associated with an increased risk of SIDS. Mitchell, A. "Results From the First Year of The New Zealand Count Death Study".

New Zealand Medical Association, 1991; 104:71-76.

Multiple Sclerosis

Although thought to be multi factorial in origin, and without a clearly defined etiology, lack of breastfeeding does appear to be associated with an increased incidence of multiple sclerosis. Dick, G., "The Etiology of Multiple Sclerosis."

Procta Royal Society of Medicine, 1976;69:611-5

Eczema

Eczema was less common and milder in babies who were breastfed (22%) and whose mothers were on a restricted diet (48%). In infants fed casein hydrolyzed, soymilk or cow's milk, 21%, 63%, and 70% respectively, developed atopic eczema. Chandra R.K., "Influence of Maternal Diet During Lactation and the Use of Formula Feed and Development of Atopic Eczema in the High Risk Infants".

British Medical Journal, 1989

Insulin Dependent Juvenile Diabetes

Cow's milk has been implicated as a possible trigger of the autoimmune response that destroys pancreatic beta cells in genetically susceptible hosts thus causing diabetes mellitus. Karjalainen, et al.,

New England Journal of Medicine - July 30, 1992

See Dr. Mark Zumhagen's *full critical Scientific Analysis* of this article on Page 95

Crohn's Disease

In this study lack of breastfeeding was a risk factor associated with later development of Crohn's disease. Koletzko, S., "Role of Infant Feeding Practices in Development of Crohn's Disease in Childhood".

British Medical Journal, 1989

Hodgkin's Disease

A statistically significant protective effect against Hodgkin's disease among children who are breastfed at least 8 months compared with children who were breastfed no more than 2 months. Schwartzbaum, J. "An Exploratory Study of Environmental and Medical Factors Potentially Related to Childhood Cancer."

Medical & Pediatric Oncology, 1991; 19(2):115-21

Delayed Development and Lower Intelligence

Lower IQ's

Children who had consumed mother's milk in early weeks of life had a significantly higher IQ at 7.5 to 8 years, than those who received no maternal milk, even after adjustment for differences between groups and mothers' educational and social class. Lucas, A., "Breast Milk and Subsequent Intelligence Quotient in Children Born Preterm".

Lancet 1992;339:261-62

Breastfed babies have slightly higher IQs than their cow-milk-fed peers. The cow does not need to have a better brain. Lendon Smith, M.D.

Let's Live, 1997

Chapter V

Vaccinations

Don't Vaccinate Before You Educate

In 1970, Robert Mendelsohn, M.D., my Pediatrics professor and godfather to my six children, was a believer in childhood immunizations. After 1970, he began to lose faith in the general value of mass immunization. In 1971, he stopped administering the Measles, Mumps, Rubella Vaccine (MMR), by 1973, he gave up on the Diphtheria, Pertussis, Tetanus Vaccine (DPT) and by 1976 he gave up on the Oral Polio Vaccine (OPV). By 1989 Dr. Mendelsohn gave up on the whole concept of vaccinations. My children's vaccine history parallels that of my late mentor. My oldest child, (born in 1971) had DPT & OPV vaccines, my next child had only OPV and my last four children, as well as my six grandchildren, have not received artificial vaccinations. My purpose is to stimulate your interest in researching further information on childhood vaccines. More and more families, after carefully weighing the evidence, are deciding not to vaccinate their children. My goal is for you to make an educated decision.

I want to raise doubt in your mind as to the safety, efficacy and moral issues of vaccines. My goal is for you to do further research into all of the vaccines, use libraries, bookstores, our internet web site (homefirst.com) and ask questions. Only after fully weighing the evidence can you make an informed decision. An informed consumer is a wise consumer. This journey is a beginning into better understanding the issues about childhood vaccinations.

ઉજઉજઉજઉજ

The following information was learned over the many years that I was a student of Dr. Mendelsohn. Also, as a practicing physician, I continued to be with Dr. Mendelsohn when he gave lectures to medical societies and university classes on his philosophy of medicine. We discussed these issues many times over the years. He later compiled much of this information into his books Confessions of a Medical Heretic and How To Raise A Healthy Child... In Spite of Your Doctor.

IMMUNIZATION AGAINST DISEASE:
A medical time bomb?

The greatest threat of childhood diseases lies in the dangerous and ineffectual efforts made to prevent them through mass immunization.

...Doctors, not politicians, have successfully lobbied for laws that force parents to immunize their children as a prerequisite for admission to school.

...They [doctors] should be nervous, because in a recent Chicago case a child damaged by a pertussis inoculation received a $5.5 million settlement award. If your doctor is in that state of mind, exploit his fear, because your child's health is at stake.

Although I administered them myself during my early years of practice, I have become a steadfast opponent of mass inoculations because of the myriad hazards they present....

Here is the core of my concern

1. There is no convincing scientific evidence that mass inoculations can be credited with eliminating any childhood disease....

2. It is commonly believed that the Salk vaccine was responsible for halting the polio epidemics that plagued American children in the 1940's and 1950's. If so, why did the epidemics also end in Europe, where polio vaccine was not so extensively used?...

3. There are significant risks associated with every immunization and numerous contraindications that may make it dangerous for the shots to be given to your child....

4. While the myriad short-term hazards of most immunizations are known (but rarely explained), no one knows the long-term consequences of injecting foreign

proteins into the body of your child. Even more shocking is the fact that no one is making any structured effort to find out.

5. There is a growing suspicion that immunization against relatively harmless childhood diseases may be responsible for the dramatic increase in autoimmune diseases since mass inoculations were introduced. These are fearful diseases such as cancer, leukemia, rheumatoid arthritis, multiple sclerosis, Lou Gehrig's disease, lupus and the Guillain-Barré syndrome....

...As a parent, only you can decide whether to reject immunizations or risk accepting them for your child. Let me urge you, though—before your child is immunized—to arm yourself with the facts about the potential risks and benefits and demand that your pediatrician defend the immunizations that he recommends.

ఇకఇకఇకఇక

WHAT'S IN A VACCINE?

Vaccines contain many ingredients of which the public is not aware. These are just some of the ingredients used to make a vaccine:

* Ethylene glycol - antifreeze

* Phenol - also known as carbolic acid. This is used as a disinfectant, dye.

* Formaldehyde - a known cancer causing agent

*Aluminum - which is associated with Alzheimer's disease and seizures also cancer producing in laboratory mice. It is used as an additive to promote antibody response.

* Thimerosal - a mercury disinfectant/ preservative. It can result in brain injury and autoimmune disease.

* Neomycin, Streptomycin - antibiotics which have caused allergic reaction in some people.

These vaccines are also grown and strained thru animal or human tissue like monkey kidney tissue, chicken embryo, embryonic guinea pig cells, calf serum, human diploid cells (the dissected organs of aborted fetuses as in the case of rubella, hepatitis A, and chicken pox vaccines)

The problem with using animal cells is that during serial passage of the virus thru the animal cells, animal RNA and DNA can be transferred from one host to another. Undetected animal viruses may slip past quality control testing procedures, as happened during the years 1955 thru 1961. The polio vaccine, which was grown on the kidney of the Green African monkey (simian), was contaminated with SV40 (simian virus #40 - the 40th discovered) which differs from the other 39 because it has oncogenic properties (cancer causing). What other viruses could be slipping by that we don't know of?

The Chicken Pox Vaccine

I was not informed that Varivax, the chicken pox vaccine, is grown on the cells of aborted fetuses until last year when one of my radio listeners sent me an article about the manufacturing process. Merck, one of the world's largest pharmaceutical companies, very cleverly uses the words "diploid tissue" instead of human tissue when they refer to the manufacturing, production and origin of the Chicken Pox Vaccine. Diploid is defined by Webster's Medical Dictionary as "having the basic chromosome number doubled". Only upon calling Merck did I find out that "diploid tissue" was human tissue. This human tissue was obtained from aborted fetuses.

Chicken pox is not necessarily a benign disease. Complications of chicken pox, in otherwise healthy children, are rare but they do occur. Chicken pox complications become even more serious in adolescents and adults [*The duration of protection of VARIVAX is unknown, at present, and the need for booster doses is not defined.*]. Among adults, chicken pox pneumonia is the most common complication, resulting in hospitalization in about one in every 400 chicken pox cases. If a vaccine could reduce the serious complications of chicken pox, ethical and moral issues aside, this vaccine may be valuable. However, Merck, in the handout that accompanies Varivax, states:

> There is insufficient data to assess the rate of
> protection of VARIVAX against the serious
> complications of chicken pox (e.g., encephalitis,
> hepatitis, pneumonitis) and during pregnancy
> (congenital varicella syndrome).
>
> Issued May 1996, Merck & Co. Inc.

In layman's terms what Merck is saying is that **their chicken pox vaccine, Varivax, does not have any proven protective effect against the serious complications of chicken pox.** Since potential complications could be one of the only medical justifications for administering the vaccine, based upon Merck's own statement, there are virtually no medical indications for the vaccine.

The purpose of a mass inoculation program is not only to lower the incidence of a disease, but more importantly to lower the serious side effects or death rates from that disease. Based on the literature distributed by Merck, the vaccinated population will either have the same serious side effects or more serious side effects. It cannot be assumed from their literature that the vaccinated population will have less serious side effects.

The following table shows a hypothetical population of 100 people, assuming more side effects in the vaccinated population with a lower incidence of diagnosed chicken pox.

EXAMPLE SHOWING MORE SERIOUS SIDE EFFECTS			
	Diagnosed with Chicken Pox	Serious Side Effects	Death from Side Effects
w/out vaccine	70%	5%	1%
with vaccine	30%	10%	2%

The following table shows a hypothetical population of 100 people, assuming the same number of side effects in the vaccinated population with a lower incidence of diagnosed chicken pox.

EXAMPLE SHOWING EQUAL SIDE EFFECTS			
	Diagnosed with Chicken Pox	Serious Side Effects	Death from Side Effects
with/out vaccine	70%	5%	1%
with vaccine	30%	5%	1%

In our hypothetical population, by using vaccinations the number of diagnosed cases may be lowered; however, the serious side effects and death rate may either be the same or greater. In the vaccinated population, these side effects and death rate may be from the natural disease, or may be a consequence of the vaccine itself.

ଓଃଔଓଃଔ

VARIVAX - The Chicken Pox Vaccine

Statements made by Merck and Co. about VARIVAX

1) Vaccination may not result in protection of all healthy, susceptible children, adolescents, and adults.
2) The duration of protection of VARIVAX is unknown at present and the need for booster doses is not defined.
3) Each dose of reconstituted vaccine contains trace quantities of neomycin (an antibiotic)

ଓଃଔଓଃଔ

Here are a few facts about VARIVAX - most of which can be found right in the manufacturers product insert.
- Individuals vaccinated with Varivax may potentially be capable of transmitting the vaccine virus to close contacts. Therefore, vaccine recipients should avoid close association with susceptible high risk individuals (e.g. newborns, pregnant women, immuno-compromised persons)
- Pregnancy should be avoided for at least 3 months after vaccination

Vaccinations

- The long term effect of administering VARIVAX Vaccine on the incidence of herpes zoster (shingles), versus those exposed to natural varicella (chicken pox) is unknown at present
- Physicians advise Varivax vaccine recipients not to use salicylates (aspirin or aspirin containing products) for six weeks after vaccination because of the chance of contracting Reyes syndrome.
- There have been no studies conducted on it for carcinogenic (cancer causing) mutagenic potential or for impairment of fertility.
- This vaccine was cultured in lung tissue obtained from two human aborted fetuses. The vaccine may even contain "residual components "of fetal lung cells.
- No one knows if this will put our children at risk for contracting chicken pox when they become older, when the complications from chicken pox can be more harmful.
- First Year of Vaccine Adverse Events Reporting System (VAERS) based surveillance of the Varicella vaccine has shown over 1,500 reports. Most of the reported categories are rashes, followed by lack of effect, fever, infections, and local injection site reactions. 5% of these reports have been serious including two deaths.

ೞೞೞೞ

Just Say No to Hepatitis B Vaccine

In December 1997, I testified against the proposal by the Illinois Department of Public Health (IDPH) to mandate hepatitis B vaccine for school children. I had already taken the course in Administrative Law in law school so I was familiar with the administration of a governmental agency. The IDPH was under no obligation to be influenced by any of the testimony presented at the hearings. Their only obligation was to hold a hearing. The passage of the mandate for compulsory hepatitis B vaccine for children would be a rubber stamp. This rubber stamping of the hepatitis B mandate did not deter the politically minded and socially conscious, consumer advocate organizations to continue to educate the public with regard to what hepatitis B disease is and to the continuing discovery of more side effects from hepatitis B vaccine.

In October of 1998 the French government ended compulsory hepatitis B vaccine in the French school system. This unique victory came about partially because of an ongoing lawsuit brought by the FNL (French National League for Liberty in Vaccination) against the government of France. Discussing the ruling of the French court in Nanterre, French Health Minister, Bernard Kouchner said "Mass inoculation of school children for hepatitis B has been stopped for fear the vaccine may produce serious neurological disorders." (i.e. Multiple Sclerosis, Chronic Fatigue Syndrome and other degenerative disorders.) In spite of this, health officers from all public health departments (State, Federal and the World Health Organization [WHO]) maintain that the vaccine was safe. The most revealing statement came from the Center for Disease Control (CDC) The CDC stated that hepatitis B vaccine "...is among the safest of vaccines". I found that to be the most revealing statement in all of the discussions and debates. The CDC alleged that the hepatitis B vaccine was among the safest vaccines. If hepatitis B vaccine is among the safest vaccines, which ones are less safe? This admission by the CDC was one of the first acknowledgments that vaccines have risks. It goes against the standard medical establishment party line, "Trust me vaccines are safe and necessary." A poll was conducted by The Chicago Sun-Times after the news release regarding the safety of the hepatitis B vaccine. The question asked was, "Do you want your child vaccinated against hepatitis B?" The results of the poll were shocking. In spite of the insistence by the CDC, WHO, IDPH, and American Academy of Pediatrics (AAP) that the hepatitis B vaccine was safe, 83% of those responding answered the question "NO". Only 17% of those who responded felt they wanted their child vaccinated with hepatitis B vaccine.

I have excerpted some of the preliminary work of Dr. Bonnie Dunbar, Professor of Cell Biology at Baylor College of Medicine (see page 125). Dr. Dunbar has been compiling data on the association between hepatitis B vaccine and Chronic Fatigue Syndrome (CFS), Multiple Sclerosis (MS) and various other auto-immune diseases. Until we get a full disclosure of the risks vs. the benefits it would be foolish to continue a program of mass vaccination. We are the greatest country in the world, partially because we are able to admit our mistakes. I have great faith that as this information about vaccines becomes more widely available, not only will the public reject vaccinations, but the scientists will eventually also reject the unscientific theory of mass immunization programs. I once again call for a moratorium on all childhood vaccinations until we assemble a consensus hearing in Washington, D.C. Let us bring the leading scientists in the related fields together. Let them present the scientific evidence with regard to vaccines. Then let them make a final determination as to the benefits vs. the risk. When presented with the evidence, those NIH Consensus Hearings said NO to fetal monitoring, NO to routine ultrasound, and NO to mammograms for women between ages 40 and 50. Until a final determination is made as to the benefits vs. the risks of vaccines, I as a father, grandfather, and physician will not advocate or administer routine vaccinations. I urge you to say "NO" to the hepatitis B vaccine.

Who is at Risk for Hepatitis B?

[Centers for Disease Control, U.S. Department of Health and Human Services, *Important Information About Hepatitis B Vaccine* 5/27/97. (Distributed by the City of Chicago, Department of Public Health.)]

1) Sexually active adults and teenagers with promiscuous lifestyles.
2) Intravenous drug abusers
3) Children born to mothers who are carriers of hepatitis B
4) Sexually active homosexual men
5) People who get tattoos, ear piercing or body piercing with unsterile needles.

 C3C3C3C3

Hepatitis B disease should not be confused with hepatitis A disease. These are two separate unique diseases with different modes of transmission. Hepatitis A can be contracted from contaminated food or contaminated water sources. Hepatitis B disease is <u>only</u> contracted from infected blood sources or sexual relations with people infected with hepatitis B. Hepatitis B is contracted from a risky lifestyle while hepatitis A is a disease which has nothing to do with lifestyle.

Hepatitis B Vaccine developed in 1987, is genetically engineered and is so new that little is known about it. It is not **even** known whether immunity will last until the babies receiving it reach an age when they might engage in high risk sexual activity or drug abuse. Yet, despite the lack of scientific evidence regarding the efficacy of hepatitis B Vaccine, the American Academy of Pediatrics, the Center for Disease Control, and the Illinois Legislature have mandated hepatitis B Vaccine for all children. Hepatitis B Vaccine is routinely given to newborns in virtually all hospitals in this country. Why the "Safe Sex Vaccine" at birth???

ଔଔଔଔ

Hepatitis B Vaccine - Professor Bonnie Dunbar

Excerpts from Professor Bonnie Dunbar, Professor of Cell Biology, Baylor College of Medicine, as posted on her web page.

Since there is a high probability that hepatitis B vaccine (or the hepatitis B virus itself) may cause MS like symptoms, Dr. Bonnie Dunbar is trying to identify more patients with autoimmune disorders that might be related to the hepatitis B vaccine in order to find a better way to prevent, diagnose, and treat such reactions.

"Within the past two years, I have had two colleagues who have developed severe and apparently permanent adverse reactions as a result of being forced to take the hepatitis B vaccine. Both of these individuals were extremely healthy and very athletic before this vaccine and have had severe, debilitating autoimmune side effects from this vaccine. I know the complete history of one, Dr. Bohn Dunbar, who is my brother who had serious rashes, joint pain, chronic fatigue and now other degenerative disorders including lupus like syndrome and multiple sclerosis like symptoms. One of my medical students went partially blind following her first booster injection and virtually completely blind in one eye following the second hepatitis B vaccine and was hospitalized for several weeks. Following two years of consulting with specialists, the consensus is that Bohn's 'syndromes' are due to adverse reactions to the hepatitis B vaccine.

I have worked in autoimmunity and vaccine development for over twenty years (the past 15 years at Baylor College of Medicine in Houston). I was honored two years ago by the National Institute of Health, as the first Margaret Pittman lecturer, for my pioneering work in contraceptive vaccines. I am, therefore, very sensitive to the balance of risk vs. benefits in vaccine development. Because of my expertise in this area, it became apparent to me that these two active, healthy individuals working in my laboratory at the same time developed "autoimmune" syndromes at the same prolonged immunological time frame following their booster injections of the hepatitis B vaccine. **After carrying out extensive literature research on this vaccine, it is apparent that the serious adverse side effects may be much more significant than generally known.** Because it is not clear that adequate long term follow-up information was collected in the clinical trial data, many of these effects might not have been observed. Even the vaccine insert, which most physicians do not show or discuss with their patients, is ominous.

I have obtained the FDA adverse reaction list of over 8,000 individuals with reported adverse reactions for the past 4 years, this covers the vaccine only. This figure does not include the Smith Kline vaccine, which I have been told includes another 15,000 or more. The vast majority of adults who have these same symptoms including rash, joint pain, chronic fatigue, neurological disorders, neuritis, rheumatoid arthritis, lupus like syndrome and multiple sclerosis like syndrome. (It has been reported by the head of the FDA that these reports indicate only about one tenth of the total numbers of adverse reactions.)

At one point a neurology specialist stated in front of myself and Bohn that 'We are having the same problem with your (Bohn's) diagnosis as we have with vets with Gulf War Syndrome who have the identical symptoms as yours--but there are no definite tests.' In reading various reports on the Gulf War Veterans illnesses, it appears that many of these symptoms are those which are related to the large numbers of adverse reactions reported for the hepatitis B vaccine. It is not clear to me, however, that this vaccine was carefully evaluated as a potential cause of some of these reactions.

CRCRCRCR

French Halt Hepatitis B Vaccine Use

Mon 05 Oct 1998 18:53:00 GMT

PARIS. Oct. 5 (UPI)

French Health Minister Bernard Kouchner says mass inoculation of school children for hepatitis B has been stopped for fear the vaccine may produce serious neurological disorders. Kouchner told French radio this morning some scientific work indicated the possibility that the vaccine might even produce cases of multiple sclerosis, or possibly augment the onset of the affliction. He said, "Problems of the central nervous system and their cause are very complicated and these possibilities must be excluded and that is why we stopped the program."

The mass immunization program began four years ago with inoculation of all 11-year-old children against hepatitis. Earlier this year, a French court in Nanterre ruled there was evidence to show a connection between the vaccine and two people with symptoms of multiple sclerosis.

...A statement from WHO officials late Friday declared the court decision could "lead to loss of public confidence in this vaccine, and decisions by other countries to suspend or delay the introduction of hepatitis B vaccine." But France has become especially prudent about such issues after disclosures its national health system failed to halt providing hemophiliacs AIDS-tainted blood products in the mid-1980s.

M.E. Comments:

Kudos to the French Government for making the wise decision eliminating the requirement for hepatitis B vaccine for school age children. Now, if only our politicians would be attentive to the findings of the French government and eliminate mandatory hepatitis B vaccine as a school requirement. When the Chicago Sun Times conducted a poll, 83% of the respondents indicated that they did not want their children vaccinated with hepatitis B vaccine.

CBCRCBCR

Chicago Sun Times
Friday, October 9, 1998

MORNINGLINE

RESULTS

Do you want your child
vaccinated against hepatitis B?

YES: 17%   NO: 83%

CBCRCBCR

Adverse Events From Vaccine Said to Outnumber Pediatric Cases of Hepatitis B

WESTPORT, Jan 25, 1999 (Reuters Health) - An advocacy group representing healthcare consumers and the vaccine-injured says that "...the number of hepatitis B vaccine-associated serious adverse event and death reports in American children under 14 outnumber the reported cases of hepatitis B disease in that age group."

The National Vaccine Information Centers calls the government-mandated policy of vaccination of all children against hepatitis B "...dangerous and scientifically unsubstantiated." The US currently mandates a 3-shot series of hepatitis B vaccinations prior to school entry. In October 1998, France ended mandatory vaccination of schoolchildren for hepatitis B because of reports of adverse events.

The organization says that in 1996, there were 872 serious hepatitis B vaccine-associated adverse events reported to the Vaccine Adverse Event Reporting System in children less than 14 years of age. Of these, 214 had received other vaccines at the same time as hepatitis B vaccination.

There were 279 cases of hepatitis B infection in children under the age of 14 in 1996.

CACACACA

Hepatitis B Statistics for All Children in U.S.A. Less than 14 Years of Age - 1996	
Cases of hepatitis B Infection	279
Serious hepatitis B vaccine adverse events	872

M.E. Comments:

The reported adverse events from hepatitis B vaccine outnumbered the number of cases of hepatitis B by three to one. It is estimated that only 15% of serious adverse reactions are actually reported. Using this percentage the actual number of serious adverse events related to hepatitis B vaccine may actually be 5,813.

03030303

FDA Bans Hepatitis B Vaccine Ingredient– Thimerosal

Actual Letters from the Internet regarding Hepatitis B Vaccine

Posted by A Mom on the Internet on January 02, 1999 at 02:52:51:

Thimerosal (a mercury derived compound) is an ingredient included in vaccines as a disinfectant and preservative. Thimerosal is also known to be a potential cause of brain injury & autoimmune disease.

IN A RULE EFFECTIVE 10-22-98, PUBLISHED IN FEDERAL REGISTER 63(77):19799-19802, 22 APRIL 1998, THE FDA BANNED USE OF MERCURY AND 15 OF IT'S COMPOUNDS, INCLUDING THIMEROSAL & MERCUROCHROME, STATING "SAFETY AND EFFECTIVE-NESS HAVE NOT BEEN ESTABLISHED FOR THE INGREDIENTS... MANUFACTURERS HAVE NOT SUBMITTED THE NECESSARY DATA."

The FDA bans Thimerosal from inclusion in over-the-counter preparations, yet considers direct injection into our children's bodies as safe and effective? This type of logic scares me, and it should scare you too!

Posted on the Internet by Interested on January 04, 1999 at 14:22:30:

In reply to: <u>FDA bans Hepatitis B Vaccine ingredient</u> posted by A Mom on January 02, 1999 at 02:52:51:
When I was researching the vaccine, My doctor provided me with the drug insert documentation for Engerix-B (the most widely administered [hepatitis B] vaccine). I read it carefully, and if I remember correctly, the ingredient that you reference was listed in its composition as a preservative. So now what ??? Can the drug companies substitute something

different, and keep selling the 'stuff', or are they considering halting the program ??? Glad we didn't do this to our kids.

ೞೲೞೲ

Posted by Robin on May 03, 1998 at 12:34:11:

I'm a registered nurse and got multiple sclerosis after my 3rd dose of hep. vac
Looking for healthcare workers noting adverse reactions to the hepatitis B vaccine. Please respond to my email. Thanks

ೞೲೞೲ

Posted by Jayne on December 10, 1998 at 01:41:30:

I went blind with severe optic neuritis within a week of hep B vac. After IV steroids some sight returned but I am still partially sighted. I am a registered nurse. I would like to know if anyone else has had a similar reaction.

ೞೲೞೲ

Posted by Alison on February 27, 1998 at 17:46:03:

I am a health care worker and have had a severe reaction to the Hep, B vaccine I have been researching it for 3 years and you are not alone there are a lot having different types of reactions and the government has added this vaccine to its adverse reaction program. Looking forward to hearing from you. Good health Robin.

ೞೲೞೲ

Vaccinations

Posted by Peter on June 09, 1998 at 13:48:08:

HFHSM.D-DM on 3 May 1998 in reply to Paula on hep B
vaccine side effects who says that because people develop
medical problems does not mean that the problem was
caused by vaccine. When a medicine or medical procedure is
administered, the symptoms experienced must been seen as
resulting from the procedure or medicine unless other insult
occurred to cause similar symptoms at the time. This is
normal medical practice. To try and tell people that their
illness was the result of something other then what actually
happened is criminal
PB

ଓଔଓଔ

Posted by Sheila on June 24, 1998 at 15:44:03:

I am 49 Yrs. Work with mentally handicapped people. In
1989 employer said that all staff needed to be vaccinated for
hep. b as we were high risk. I did not know what hepatitis B
was. Employer said that the vaccine was completely safe
because it was man made, it did not have any of the
hepatitis virus in it. The day after the vaccination I was very
ill. Could not walk with pains all over body. Employer said
that illness was not related to vaccine. Since that time my
health has been very bad. Constant infections. Always tired,
feel more like 90 then 49. No longer able to play golf, take
pictures, enjoy sex. I have recently been diagnosed as having
chronic fatigue syndrome. I am in consultation with

solicitors and am trying to take legal action against my employer.

ⳤⳤⳤⳤ

Posted by Mary Ann on November 22, 1998 at 12:45:48:

Have had severe fatigue, increased sleeping, abdominal discomfort, muscle and joint pain, head-aches and bloating. This is aside from the chronic active hepatitis C I have. I have very severe symptoms i.e. fatigue, muscle, joint and abdominal pain and other. I received the first of the series of the hepatitis A and B vaccines last Tuesday and the above (1st set) of symptoms developed overnight. I can barely move. I hope it wears off.

ⳤⳤⳤⳤ

Flu Vaccine

In 1976, when I just started in my medical practice, one of the great experiments in "modern" medicine took place. The Center for Disease Control predicted a devastating flu epidemic, the "Swine Flu" epidemic. They predicted that thousands of people would die from this strain of flu just as in the flu epidemic of 1918 which caused the deaths of millions of Americans. In order to **"protect"** the American people from this "certain death" the government made the Swine Flu vaccine available free of charge to the public and began administering it at "government vaccine centers". I asked my professor, the late Dr. Robert Mendelsohn, "what should I recommend to my patients, if the government makes this vaccine mandatory?" His response was, "Tell your patients to line up at the back of the line and pray that they run out of vaccine material before your patients reach the front of the line." After just a few weeks, almost 100 people died shortly after being injected with the Swine Flu vaccine and more than 500 people developed Guillain-Barré syndrome (GBS) (see explanation following). The government immediately abandoned the Swine Flu vaccine program. As for the prediction that thousands of people would die from the flu, the total number of cases of Swine

Flu was less than 10. This is not the first time that the
government and our medical establishment have tried to
scare the public into accepting unproven medical
treatments. It is no different with hospital birth, bottle
feeding, antibiotics, surgery, etc. The argument is always
the same, the medical establishment says, "If you do not
follow my advice, very bad things will happen to you. Trust
me, I am your doctor." The time has come to say, "show me
the evidence, show me that the treatment is safer than the
disease." Let us get back to this principle of Hippocrates,
the father of medicine, "Primum Non Nocere - Above all do
no harm," a principle that medicine violates over and over
again.

It is my interpretation, according to medical statistics,
that the flu vaccine of today is no safer than the Swine Flu
vaccine of 1976. The only difference is that in 1976 the flu
vaccine was administered to thousands of individuals at
government vaccine centers and the data relating to the side
effects was readily available. Today, the vaccine is
administered in thousands and thousands of doctors offices,
work places, drug stores, and grocery stores, with no
uniform methodology for reporting accountability or follow
up data easily available. Therefore, serious side effects,
such as Guillain-Barré Syndrome, are easily missed and the
connection is never made. The evidence is not conclusive
that the risk of the flu vaccine outweighs the alleged benefits
(saving thousands of lives). However, the evidence seems to

show that the flu vaccine does have some very serious side effects.

At this time, we need to call for a moratorium on all vaccinations. We need to convene a panel of the leading experts in medicine. This panel must be devoid of sponsorship from any drug companies or parties that have any vested interest in the outcome. The panel should review all the scientific articles and data on vaccinations. Afterwards, they should make their recommendations. It is very interesting that whenever the National Institute of Health has convened such consensus panels the results are far different than we would expect. In the past, these NIH consensus panels have recommended fewer ultra sounds, fewer breast cancer surgeries, less cesarean sections, and they have questioned routine mammograms for women. I have great faith in the honesty of scholarly physicians. When they meet in large consensus groups and review data they come to unbiased conclusions relying on the information presented to them and not relying on political agendas, or their own beliefs.

At the present time, your doctor will try to scare you about the flu, until all the evidence is in, Mayer Eisenstein, M.D., will scare you about the flu vaccine. My advice is say "No" to the flu vaccine. If you get the flu ask your grandmother for her chicken soup recipe!

The following information was learned over the many years that I was a student of Dr. Mendelsohn. See page 112.

"The mad vehemence of Modern Medicine is nowhere more evident than in the yearly influenza vaccine farce. I can never think about flu shots without remembering a wedding I once attended. Strangely enough, no grandparents were among the participants and no one seemed to be over age 60. When I finally asked where all the old folks were, I was told they had all received their flu shots a few days before. They were all at home recovering from the shots' ill effects!

The entire flu shot effort resembles some massive roulette game, since from one year to the next it's anybody's guess whether the strains immunized against will be the strains that are epidemic. We were all afforded a peek at the real dangers of flu vaccines when in 1976, the Great Swine Flu Fiasco revealed, under close government and media surveillance, 565 cases of Guillain-Barré paralysis resulting from the vaccine and thirty "unexplained" deaths of older persons within hours after receiving the shot. I wonder what would be the harvest of disaster if we kept as close a watch on the effects of all the other flu shot campaigns. Dr. John Seal, of the National Institute of Allergy and Infectious Disease says, "We have to go on the basis that any and all flu vaccines are capable of causing Guillain-Barré syndrome."

ᘒᘓᘒᘓᘒᘓ

ONE FLU OVER THE CUCKOO'S NEST

http://www.4icpa.org/research/vaccinat.htm

"Vaccine enthusiasts reached the height of their folly in 1976 when a pandemic of "killer Swine Flu" was predicted. America was asked to buy a "pig in a poke" and accept vaccination. The media proclaimed that failure to do so would result in an epidemic that would rival any in recorded history. The government spent millions on the vaccine. The outcome: There were deaths. There were cases of paralysis, but they were not from the dreaded "killer flu." They resulted from the vaccine that was supposed to prevent it.

J. Anthony Morris, one time head of influenza control in the U.S. warned his superiors in the federal government that the vaccine was dangerous and probably ineffective. When they refused to act, he went directly to the media. Morris advised the public that the vaccine was unsafe, and an epidemic was unlikely. As a result, he was fired from his position at the Food and Drug Administration. His experimental animals, representing years of research, were destroyed. Publication of his findings was blocked by his superiors.

Other scientists and physicians were also critical of the vaccine. Nobel Laureate, Linus Pauling, in a letter to the first author dated May 11, 1976, indicated that he and his wife did not intend to take the vaccine because he felt there was "significant dangers" associated with it. The Lancaster, Pennsylvania *Intelligencer Journal* of August 14, 1976 reported on a survey of practicing physicians asked about the vaccine. 100 percent of the physicians surveyed said they would not administer Swine Flu shots to their own children. T.A. Vonder Haar, then Coordinator of Programs in Public Policy at the University of Missouri, stated in a letter dated May 10, 1976. "Virus vaccines are notoriously ineffective...flu vaccines have been documented as having contained SV.40, a known carcinogen, with full FDA knowledge."

Even the insurance industry balked at this one. They refused to indemnify vaccine makers against claims arising from the administration of Swine Flu vaccine. C. Joseph Stetler, then president of the Pharmaceutical Manufacturer's Association was quoted by UPI as saying, "It's like you taking out a life insurance policy and suddenly becoming a kamikaze pilot." The answer — the government agreed to insure the vaccine makers! What was the result of this debacle?

According to Newsweek, July 18, 1977, $135 million was appropriated by Congress to indemnify vaccine makers. However, claims totaling over $1.3 billion dollars were filed with the Justice Department alleging injury or death as a result of the Swine Flu shots. 517 Americans were stricken with Guillain-Barré syndrome, and at least 23 died. And what of the killer epidemic? The total number of Swine Flu cases was six, and in some cases the diagnosis was questionable.

Are things better today? A common ritual in America is getting a flu shot "just in case" when "flu season" is imminent. How safe and effective are today's influenza vaccines? Scheifle et. al. in a study reported in the *Canadian Medical Association Journal,* January 15, 1990, described the results of hospital workers receiving trivalent influenza vaccine prepared for the 1988-1989 flu season...

"Of approximately 500 full-time workers in 'high risk' areas, 288 took the vaccine. Of these, 266 returned a questionnaire regarding any symptoms experienced within 48 hours after the vaccination. 90 percent of the respondents reported adverse effects. 49 percent reported systemic adverse effects. Five percent missed work as a consequence of vaccine adverse effects."

CRURUR

Guillain-Barré Syndrome

Guillain-Barré (*ghee yan-bah ray*) **Syndrome**, (**GBS**) is a rare and unpredictable syndrome which causes the person's life to go into utter chaos and turmoil. This syndrome, is also called ***acute idiopathic polyneuritis***, a disorder that consists of weakness and even paralysis of many of the body's muscles, along with abnormal sensations. The illness can be present in several ways, at times making the diagnosis difficult to establish in its early stages. The specific cause is not known. Research to date indicates that, the nerves of the person who has Guillain-Barré, are attacked by the body's defense system against disease (antibodies and white blood cells). As a result of this attack, the nerve insulation (myelin) and sometimes even the covered conducting part of the nerve (axon) is damaged. This causes delay or change of the nerve "messages", between the sender (usually the brain, cortex or spinal column) and receiver (usually a muscle). The abnormal sensations and weakness quickly follow.

CSCECSCR

Judge loses use of hands, legs

Chicago Sun Times - Wed., February 4, 1998

"The chief judge of Will County Circuit Court has been diagnosed with Guillain-Barré syndrome, an illness that has left him unable to use his hands and legs.

Herman Hasse, 55, became ill two weeks ago while attending a judicial conference in Miami.

Hasse had flu-like symptoms before leaving and family members told him the illness might have been triggered by a flu shot. The Illinois Department of Health said there is no statistically significant risk of getting the syndrome from a flu shot."

಄಄಄಄

GBS and Flu Shot
Responses posted on the Internet:
Submitted by Teresa on 6/30/98.

Would like to know about death from GBS, 2 wk incubation period from flu shot, symptoms, etc. my dad just died mysteriously, had many symptoms of GBS, but had recently had a flu shot. His immune system was very poor, overall physical and mental health was poor.

಄಄಄಄

Submitted by Doris on 2/22/98.

My husband and I were told 2 things:

1 - The neurologist and immunologist who treated Steve told him that they would personally never get another vaccine if they were him UNLESS it was life threatening.

2 - At a MD Chapter meeting in Nov '97, Dr Carol Koski, head of Neurology at Univ of MD, was asked about the flu shot and GBS. She said GBS patients should refrain from getting the flu shot for one year after getting GBS. After that, she saw no reason why the annual flu shot couldn't be resumed.

On a personal basis, my husband Steve came down with GBS in '96 - in Oct '95 he rec'd his first flu shot. In Jan '96 he rec'd a cocktail of shots for an overseas trip. Could there be a connection ?

છ૦૨૦૩૦૨

Submitted by Steve on 5/24/98.

I got GBS in 1981 shortly after taking the flu shot. I never took the shot again for years. I finally decided to take the flu shot again in the mid-90's. I think I took it two or three times with no GBS. But, in '96, I took the shot and soon thereafter developed a bad rash on my abdomen. A short time later, I developed GBS again. I am not sure if the rash was connected, but I am personally convinced that the flu shot and GBS are connected in my case. I will never take the shot again, and my neurologist agreed.

છ૦૨૦૩૦૨

A Personal Story Guillain Barré After Flu Vaccine as posted on the Internet.

Ray's story...

Wife Martha & I had experienced flu attacks in January 1994 & 1995. Nothing severe - just put us to bed except to get up for something to eat once each day for about a week. Low-grade fever, aching, continuing cough, etc. However, there are more pleasant things so we decided in the fall of '95 to undergo the flu shot - neither of us had had one for at least 40 years. I was 63 and retired. Have had blood pressure problems for 25 years & some heart arrhythmia, but no general symptoms and pretty much do as I wish (had never been hospitalized a day in my life).. We both received one injection of Parke-Davis' "Fluogen" vaccine. Were told to come for a second one in two weeks since it had been so long since being vaccinated. Neither of us have returned for that second shot, nor will we ever do so.

I assume we were given vaccine from the same vial. I went first and noticed the nurse agitating the vial. I could see thru the liquid against the backlight of the fridge interior light and noticed some light particulate moving thru the liquid. I know some vaccines appear this way & was not concerned. Martha was injected in the upper left arm and had some soreness for several days. My injection was to the upper left muscle on top of the shoulder. The only effect I noted was the other shoulder muscle was a little sore the next day. The shots were given on 9/21/95. Martha had no further problems. On 10/1/95 I awoke with everything tasting as if I had a mouthful of salt. This went on all day. On the morning of 10/2/95 I noticed that everything tasted bad (no longer salty). Even water tasted strange. Later I went to the bathroom to wash my hands and started in cold water - it felt hot. When it warmed to lukewarm it was excruciating. Carpal tunnel syndrome had returned to my wrists. This had not bothered during the seven years since my retirement. Later that afternoon I went to check the mailbox feeling okay, but was so weak on the return trip I barely made it back into the house. Never mind - all will be well tomorrow.

On the morning of 10/3/95 Martha had to pull me out of bed. I could not get to a sitting position even by extending my legs over the side of the bed and using them as a counter-weight. Went to the bathroom to prepare for a doctor visit and somehow wound up on the floor unable to get up. With my arms extended backward behind me and bouncing on my backside I managed to get to the den. By placing my hands on the low couch behind me and pushing hard with my feet & legs was able to get to a setting position on the couch. As I dressed Martha pulled the car across the sidewalk just beyond the porch & left the door open. With my hands on her shoulders, I was able to rise from the couch and follow her to the car.

Having called in advance the doctor's office met me with a wheelchair. Wheeled into an examining room, first check was blood pressure - over the moon. Had tried to check it the night before but could not get my machine pumped high enough to get a systolic (upper) reading & assumed the machine was broken. They immediately arranged a hospital room (just across the driveway) & I was wheeled over & checked in.

Two days of testing which included blood work-ups, urinalyses, X-rays, CAT scan & MRI I was finally diagnosed with a spinal tap which revealed high protein in the spinal fluid. Evaluation was AIDP & it was on to ICU. About the third day in ICU my breathing declined & I was ventilated. In the 30 days in ICU (15 with the ventilator in place) I would estimate my conscious time at not more than 2 hours and that was marginal. I was pronounced paraplegic at one point, being able to move only my toes very slightly. Plasmapheresis (plasma exchange) did nothing for me. However, three small infusions of IVIG (intravenous immunoglobulin) & body movement returned. A fourth infusion did very little and the fifth was canceled. I came to in Rehab a day later with some slight paralysis to both hands but was told I would be unable to walk. In my first trip to Physical Therapy I could not even rise to stand on the parallel bars (too weak from 30 days with no food other than albumin 5% on the IV. However, on the second day I rose & walked the length of the bars. Two days later I was on the walker and I walked from the hospital without aid on the 21st day of Rehab. I am left with feet which still feel stiff (they are not), good walking ability on smooth surfaces (not so good on rough or slanted terrain), hands that are sometimes a little stiff and tingle, as do the feet. In ICU I encountered blood pressures in the high 200's and as low as 34 (deadly). I encountered 5 blood clots which had to be dissolved and had a vena cava filter installed to catch any clot fragments which entered the bloodstream. This will remain for the balance of my life.

Guillain-Barré Syndrome is a dangerous, potentially deadly condition with long-term after effects. Persons contemplating the influenza shot should be made aware that this is an always present possibility, and need to realize that GBS is not some mild reaction, but is rather a hard paralysis capable of bringing on disability, severe illness and death.

ℭℬℭℬℭℬℭℬ

"Revaccinations Not Necessary After Flu Vaccine Recall"

OLYMPIA, Wash.--February 13, 1997-- Parke-Davis today recalled all remaining lots of its Fluogen influenza due to a decrease in potency.

The vaccine was recalled after tests conducted by Parke-Davis showed that the potency of the vaccine was decreasing, and may not adequately protect recipients against the strains of influenza that had been seen this season.

M.E. Comments:

However, the ineffectiveness of the Fluogen influenza vaccine to protect against influenza, did not prevent Ray from developing GBS.

ℭℬℭℬℭℬℭℬ

The Flu Vaccine Is It Really Safe and Effective?
What Is In A Flu Vaccine?

Formaldehyde: a known cancer causing agent
Thimerosal: (a mercury derivative) used as a preservative in the vaccine, can cause brain injury and autoimmune disease.   Also this vaccine is propagated on chicken embryo cells.

The problem with using animal cells is that during serial passage of the virus thru the animal cells, animal RNA and DNA can be transferred from one host to another. Undetected animal viruses may slip past quality control testing procedures (see page 115).

In 1995 a team of Swiss scientists discovered an enzyme, reverse transcriptase. Keep in mind reverse transcriptase copies RNA and DNA and is associated with retroviruses in MMR vaccines and some influenza vaccines that had been propagated in chicken embryo .

ෆෂෆෂ

How Effective is the Vaccine?

Flu vaccine production is a big guessing game. Every year the CDC has to try and predict what virus will infect people in the U.S. the following year. This is something like looking thru a crystal ball. So how accurate is this crystal ball?

In 1992-93 the isolated influenza samples for the predominant virus (influenza A (H3N2) virus) were not similar to that in the vaccine (MMWR 42 752-55).

In the 1994-95 influenza season the CDC reported that 43% of isolated influenza samples for the predominant virus were not similar to the vaccine. The same goes for another type A virus (HINI) and the influenza B they also were not similar to that in the vaccine (MMWR 9/8/95).

In a 1993 Dutch article on a nursing home for the elderly, 50% of the vaccinated population contracted the illness compared to 48% of the unvaccinated.

Vaccine efficiency in elderly is usually never higher then 52-67%. Other doctors and studies declare it even lower, showing an efficiency rate of 20% or less and if you keep in mind mistakes in production, transport, and storage this may even cause a further decrease in effectiveness.

ଔଔଔଔ

How Safe are Flu Vaccines?
We have all heard of the Swine Flu vaccine disaster of 1976 that left over 565 cases of Guillain-Barré Syndrome paralysis, as well as other neurological problems and many unexplained deaths among recently vaccinated elderly.

Although vaccine manufacturers try to say today's vaccines do not carry the same risk of Guillain Barré Syndrome as with the Swine Flu vaccine, many cases (as well as other neurological problems) are still occurring after flu vaccines. In the early 1980's Dr. John Seal of the National Institute of Allergy and Infectious Disease stated that "We have to go on the basis that any and all flu vaccines are capable of causing Guillain- Barré."

Flu vaccine product inserts do state that individuals who have a history of Guillain-Barré syndrome have a substantially greater likelihood of subsequently developing GBS.

In 1970, G.A. Rosenberg, in an article in the New England Journal of Medicine, wrote about meningoencephalitis being reported as a result of influenza vaccines. He then goes on to describe a case of a patient in which meningoencephalitis developed 12 days after vaccination with a purified influenza vaccine.

Other reactions that have been associated with past influenza vaccines are: fever, malaise, myalgia, hives, angioedema, allergic asthma, systemic anaphylaxis, Guillain- Barré Syndrome, encephalopathy, optic neuritis, brachial plexus neuropathy, many different types of paralysis, myletitis polyneuritis (including cases of polyradiculitis, polyradiculomyelitis, and polyganglioradiculitis), ataxia, respiratory infections, gastro-intestinal problems, eye problems, allergic thrombocytopenia, disturbed blood pressure, collapse, etc.

ೞೞೞೞ

Vaccinations

REFERENCES

Center For Complex Infectious Diseases -
http://www.ccid.org/
John Martin, M.D., Ph.D. - Web Site
This site provides information on stealth viruses. The
issue of live viral vaccines as a probable source of
certain stealth viruses and a known source of SV40 virus
is also addressed.

Centers for Disease Control and Prevention -
http://www.cdc.gov/ncidod/diseases/flu/fluvac.htm

Concerned Parents for Vaccine Safety's Home Page -
http://home.sprynet.com:80/sprynet/Gyrene/

Department of Neurology at Massachusetts General Hospital
http://neuro-www.mgh.harvard.
edu/forum/GuillainBarreSyndromeMenu.html

GBS Syndrome -
http://terri.adsnet.com/jsteinhi/html/gbs/gbsmain.html

Hepatitis B Vaccine Study -
http://webpages.netlink.co.nz/~ias/dunbar.htm
Dr. Bonnie S. Dunbar, PhD, Professor, Department of
Cell Biology Baylor College of Medicine, has identified
patients with autoimmune disorders that might be
related to the hepatitis B vaccine in order to find a better
way to prevent, diagnose, and treat such reactions.
Since it is clearly established that this vaccine (or the
virus infection itself) may cause multiple sclerosis like

symptoms, further information could be a great help for her ongoing research.

How Safe Is Universal Hepatitis B Vaccination? - **www.waisbrenclinic.com**
Burton A. Waisbren, Sr., M.D., F.A.C.P. - Web Site
In this scholarly paper Dr. Waisbren discusses four of the theories with regard to the association between hepatitis B vaccine and adverse neurological findings (i.e. multiple sclerosis, chronic fatigue syndrome, Guillain-Barré, etc.)

ILLINOIS VACCINE AWARENESS COALITION (IVAC)
P.O. Box 946, Oak Park, IL 60303
Phone: (708) 848-0116
Barbara Alexander Mularkey
Call or write for outstanding information on vaccines.

Mendelsohn, Robert S. M.D., How To Raise A Healthy Child... In Spite of Your Doctor, Contemporary Books, Inc., Chicago.

Mendelsohn, Robert S. M.D., Confessions of a Medical Heretic, 1979, Contemporary Books.

National Vaccine Information Center (NVIC) - **http://www.909shot.com/**
An outstanding site for information on vaccinations. A must!

Ohio Parents for Vaccine Safety
251 West Ridgeway Drive, Dayton, OH 45459
Phone: (937) 435-4750
Christine M. Severyn, R.Ph., Ph.D., Director

Vaccinations

Call or write for outstanding newsletters on vaccines, as well as complimentary information.

Vaccine Information & Awareness -
http://www.access1.net/via/
VIA empowers parents to question, challenge, investigate, research, and become more informed and aware about the risks and dangers that exist with vaccines.

Tetrahedron -
www.tetrahedron.org
Dr. Len Horowitz - Web Site
This web site will be of interest to all those who want to be better informed of the risks of childhood vaccines. Dr. Horowitz points the finger at contaminated vaccines as a potential cause of AIDS, Ebola, Asthma, Chronic fatigue, Depression, Colitis, Diabetes, Breast Cancer, Prostate Cancer, and others.

Vaccination? The Choice is Yours! -
http://www.avn.org.au/
"In light of the high public regard for medicine, it may come as a surprise that modern medical techniques such as vaccinations and antibiotics have had no significant impact on the overall death rate in industrialized societies during the past century. Death rates in these societies have certainly declined sharply - but they did so before the introduction of vaccinations and antibiotics."

www.homefirst.com - go to vaccine links.

Chapter VI

Antibiotics

Ear Infections and Antibiotics
One Grandmother is Worth Two Pediatricians.
If your child develops an ear infection should
you treat with antibiotics???

The answer in the past was a resounding **yes**! However, there is mounting scientific evidence that not only are antibiotics the wrong treatment, but they can lead to problems such as recurrent ear infections, hearing loss, as well as total systemic resistance to more serious types of infections.

Isn't it strange that anti-histamines, given to children with a common cold, can actually prolong statis of the fluid in the middle ear and can actually increase the incidence of bacterial ear infection? Isn't it strange that many of the newer generation antibiotics used by pediatricians in the treatment of ear infections may cause hearing loss?? Isn't it strange that Tympanostomy Tubes (tubes put in the ears to prevent ear infections) may actually cause hearing loss??? Isn't it strange that most ear infections start at two months of age, approximately the same time that the first series of vaccines are introduced????

My late mentor, Robert S. Mendelsohn, M.D. once said "one grandmother is worth two pediatricians," so my modern day "scientific" answer is to replace your pediatrician with a grandmother. My grandmother used remedies like warm olive oil, hot water bottle, and massive amounts of TLC for the treatment of ear infections. Not only are these methods effective, but unlike antibiotics they do not start a cycle of repeat ear infections.

There are only three answers to reduce the **24,500,000** ear infections that are prevalent in our country (virtually all of which are treated unnecessarily with antibiotics) – breastfeeding, breastfeeding and more breastfeeding. This will prevent approximately 22 million of the ear infections. The remaining ones should be treated with your grandmother and my grandmother's remedies. Yes, I am saying that until your pediatrician follows the scientific evidence he/she should play no part in the treatment of ear infections.

೫೦೩೦೩೦೩

Dr. Larry Culpepper, in an article in "Journal of the American Medical Association" 1997; 278: 1643-1645, writes that...

"Evidence that routine antimicrobial treatment improves the course and outcome after acute otitis media is weak. Given the lack of evidence for benefit and the potential for adverse affects, ...routine treatment using 10 days of antimicrobials for all cases of acute otitis media is not warranted. ...Since evidence that microbials are effective therapy for otitis media is lacking, it is not surprising that neither type nor duration of administration [2 days, 5 days, 7 days or 10 days] has been shown to affect outcomes. ...Increasing world wide bacterial resistance to antimicrobials is responsible for added morbidity, mortality and costs. The most frequent outpatient use of antimicrobials is for otitis media, with the number of prescriptions increasing from almost 12 million in 1980 to almost 23.6 million in 1992."

ଔଔଔଔ

In the "Journal of Pediatrics" 1998; 101 Number 1. Dr. Dowell, et al, writes that...

"Otitis media is the leading indication for outpatient antimicrobial use in the United States. Over diagnosis of and unnecessary prescribing for this position has contributed to the spread of antimicrobial resistance." [The goal will be to] avoid up to 8 million unnecessary courses of antibiotics annually. Criteria for defining these conditions ...as well as the evidence supporting deferring antibiotic treatment [are presented]. Discussions of shortened courses of antibiotics for acute otitis media and restricted indication for antimicrobial prophylaxis are also presented."

❧❧❧❧

In "Pediatrics" 1999; 103: 395-398 Dr. Bauchner, in a shameful admission that doctors do not practice evidence based scientific medicine, states that...

"More than half of the physicians surveyed believed that parental pressure contributed most to antibiotic overuse."

❧❧❧❧

In *British Medical Journal* 2000; 320: 350-354, Dr. Roger Damoiseaux concludes that...

"Prescription of Amoxicillin at the first visit improves symptomatic outcome in only 1 of every 7-8 children younger than 2 years of age with acute otitis media...

On the other hand, antibiotic treatment did not affect the duration of pain or crying in young children, did not have any significant effect on clinical symptoms, and did not improve tympanometry findings at six weeks, compared with placebo.... These results do not justify the routine prescription of Amoxicillin to all children aged younger than 2 years with acute otitis media..."

ᏣᏇᏣᏇ

"Pediatrics" Vol 102; 1998: No. 1 In an editorial commentary on "Ways to Reduce Inappropriate Oral Antibiotic Use" Drs. Bauchner and Philipp stated...

"There is increasing concern in the medical community about inappropriate antibiotic use. ...[Therefore] the American Academy of Pediatrics *Redbook* has changed its recommendation for empiric antibiotic therapy for life-threatening infections in which the pneumococcus is a possible etiologic agent. ...Unfortunately we have spent the last four decades convincing the public that antibiotics are miracle drugs

...A realistic claim because they save lives and reduce morbidity. However, times and disease have changed. We now must reeducate ourselves and our patients about the appropriate role that antibiotics play in the health of children."

ᏣᏇᏣᏇ

Dr. Alfred Berg, a Professor of Family Medicine at the University of Washington recommends that you talk to your doctor before demanding or accepting drugs as a preventative measure against acute ear infections...

"There is no good scientific evidence indicating that low-dose prophylactic use of antibiotics is effective at reducing ear infections in most kids."

ભહ્યભહ્ય

Parenting magazine, March 1997, reported that a Federal panel convened to study treatments of otitis media (ear infection) found that a wait and see approach may be the best medicine. In about 95% of cases the panel found, the ear fluid goes away on its own and there is virtually no evidence that children suffer long term hearing loss as a result of otitis media.

ભહ્યભહ્ય

In *Family Practice News*, March 15, 1993 it was reported...

"Physicians need to hang tough when they are hammered by their young patients' parents and their surgical colleagues to place Tympanostomy tubes in children with recurrent otitis or persistent middle ear effusions (fluid in the ear). Accumulating evidence shows this treatment can lead to hearing loss down the line."

ભહ્યભહ્ય

Pediatrics, May 1993, vol. 91, p. 86, reported that...

"In a presentation on infant and childhood acute otitis and middle ear effusions, Dr. Heinz Eichenwald, William Buchanan Professor of Pediatrics at the University of Texas Southwestern Medical School in Dallas, challenged the prevailing medical opinion in support of tube placement with some fairly recent studies, and he urged family physicians to consider the finding carefully before they recommend insertion of tubes in the future.

Dr. Eichenwald set out to find similar accounts in the literature. A Scandinavian investigation showed, even in children who had the tubes removed one year after insertion, hearing loss continued to occur for as long as twelve years. "This seemingly harmless procedure does something to the ear" Dr. Eichenwald, asserted to the annual meeting of the California Academy of Family Physicians."

ΣΟΣΟΣΟΣΟ

In *Family Practice News,* August 1, 1992, it was reported that...

Infants who were breast-fed exclusively for at least four months had significantly fewer cases of otitis media than those who had not been breast-fed exclusively; this protective effect remained after potential confounding factors were controlled. The reasons for this protective effect are unknown, but they may include immunologic properties of breast milk or the differences in position while nursing and bottle feeding. The authors conclude that breast feeding for four or more months provides a protective effect against otitis media.

Oral decongestants, with or without antihistamines, add nothing to the treatment of otitis media or sinusitis in children, Dr. Heinz Eichenwald said at the annual meeting of the Kansas Academy of Family Physicians. When given to the child with a common cold, these agents may actually prolong the effusion in the middle ear and increase the incidence of a bacterial otitis, said Dr. Eichenwald, of the University of Texas Southwestern Medical Center at Dallas. The best decongestant to use is warm steam. "We have nothing that works more effectively in the child. It should really be a part of the treatment" of otitis media, sinusitis, and common colds, he said.

M.E. Comments:

How many scientific studies will be necessary until pediatricians get it? Ear infection does not equal antibiotics. What a bunch of hogwash, that physicians are pressured by parents to prescribe antibiotics. Why are these same physicians not pressured into home birth, breastfeeding, natural progesterone cream, no vaccinations, etc.? The only treatments that physicians are pressured into are the ones that they believe in, irrespective of the scientific evidence. How shameful!!

ೞೞೞೞ

REFERENCES

Bauchner and Philipp, Editorial "Ways to Reduce Inappropriate Oral Antibiotic Use". <u>Pediatrics</u> Vol 102; 1998: No. 1

Bauchner, Dr.,"Pediatrics" 1999; 103: 395-398.

Culpepper, Dr. Larry, "Journal of the American Medical Association" 1997; 278: 1643-1645.

Damoiseaux, Dr. Roger, <u>British Medical Journal</u> 2000; 320: 350-354.

Dowell, et al, "Journal of Pediatrics" 1998; 101 Number 1.

<u>Pediatrics</u>, May 1993, vol. 91, p. 86.

Chapter VII

Ritalin
The Drugging of Our Children

In 1971, I was a third year medical student at the
University of Illinois. Ritalin, a drug which acts as a
stimulant in adults, was marketed to children who were
labeled as hyperactive. The drug, allegedly, had minimal
side effects and reduced the effects of hyperactivity. In
1972, Dr. Robert Mendelsohn, together with the National
Health and Environmental Law Program, petitioned the
Food & Drug Administration to withdraw approval of Ritalin
for use in children. The petition alleged that Ritalin was
both unsafe and ineffective. The FDA denied the petition
stating that the evidence showed that Ritalin was both safe
and effective. At the same time that doctors were discussing
the effectiveness and safety of Ritalin, one of my classmates
had published a letter to the editor in the New England
Journal of Medicine discussing the nature of the abuse of
Ritalin. It seems that the pediatricians were the last people
to admit how addictive and dangerous Ritalin had become.
During the 1970's approximately 200,000 children were
being treated with Ritalin for alleged hyperactivity. As the
1970's came to an end, the number of children being treated
with Ritalin had not substantially changed. Naively, I
believed that as doctors became educated as to the dangers

of Ritalin and the elusive nature of the diagnosis of "hyperactivity," the use of Ritalin would decrease. How wrong I was! ! !

With the financial backing of the pharmaceutical giant Ciba-Geigy, the drug company which produces Ritalin, use of Ritalin soared from 200,000 in the 1970's to 1,000,000 children in 1986 and has reached almost 4,000,000 children today.

Scientific studies have documented: the sudden death caused by Ritalin; the abnormal brain functions caused by Ritalin; the growth suppression caused by Ritalin; the neurological tics caused by Ritalin; agitation, addiction and psychosis caused by Ritalin. The March 18, 1996 cover story of Newsweek magazine was "Ritalin Are We Over medicating Our Kids?" and the November 30, 1998 cover of Time magazine was "The Latest on Ritalin - Scientists last week said it works. But how do you know if it's right for your kids?" Also, there have been more than ten well documented books on the dangers of Ritalin.

How many more of our children will have to be exposed to dangerous drugs, such as Ritalin, prescribed by our pediatricians and psychiatrists before we "wake up"? While, in some instances, attention deficit disorder does exist, the treatment is not a dangerous drug, whose side effects rival those of cocaine. If your child's doctor recommends Ritalin, it is time for you to do some serious research into alternative treatments. If your school will not allow your child to continue unless he/she is placed on Ritalin, it is time to look for alternative forms of education (maybe private schooling, home schooling etc.). **Today Ritalin, tomorrow Prozac, and the next day Viagra????**

CACACA

Robert F. Willey, Chicago, IL, University of Illinois Medical School wrote in *The New England Journal of Medicine,* August 19, 1971, page 464, on "ABUSE OF METHYLPHENIDATE (RITALIN)"...

"*To the Editor:* Being extremely interested in the discussion and debate taking place among professional and lay people in this country over the problem of drug abuse, I wish to submit the following observations.

I am working this summer at the only accredited prison hospital in the country — Cermak Memorial Hospital—at the House of Corrections in Chicago, and I have been administering the drug-abuse program while the regular nurse is on vacation. Recently, I received several reports from the men on the program that there is a new thing turning on their particular micro society. Their term is "West Coast." Many have at least tried it, and an increasing number are becoming addicted to it.

I was informed by one prisoner who has a 20-year-old heroin habit that he mainlined "West Coast" just once and that he was finding himself "running" (the vernacular for trying to put it on the street) for it. The same man told me that it is not covered by the drug-abuse laws. A second inmate, who is an addict both to heroin and to "West Coast" but mostly to "West Coast," told me today that in the two months that he was out of jail he lost 14 kg (30 pounds) and got little or no sleep (he also has the abscess problems that virtually all these men have from "shooting" quinine and using dirty needles). He is nervous and jittery and seeks only more "West Coast" to keep him going.

One of the main reasons I am writing this letter is that all the prisoners I have talked to about this increasing problem got the drug with a doctor's prescription. Many of them are getting it with their aid privileges and selling what they don't use to earn money to support themselves and their habit. This menacing drug is being released to these men by careless physicians, who, I hope, will read this letter and act on the knowledge I am trying to impart.

The more proper name for "West Coast" is methylphenidate, or perhaps doctors know it as Ritalin. Yes, it is the most highly addicting and dangerous drug that any of these men can think of, and they have had much clinical experience in the matters of intravenous addiction."

⊰⊱⊰⊱

Guardian magazine quoting Thomas Szasz, M.D., author of <u>Manufacture of Madness</u>, on December 22, 1971 writes...

"I consider the characterization of hyperactivity in children, in the absence of objectively demonstrable evidence of neurological malfunctioning, so absurd as not to deserve to be taken seriously. The labeling of such children as ill is a social strategy to justify controlling them by means of drugs.

The use of Ritalin for school children may be a "social strategy," but profit is behind it, too. A new children's market has opened up and CIBA has it cornered. According to reports, Ritalin is bringing in 15% of CIBA's gross profits, or $13 million a year. Barring widespread protest by masses of people, the market for the drug has hardly been tapped."

⊰⊱⊰⊱

USA Today - November 16, 1995, reported that Gene Halslip, the Drug Enforcement Administration's Head of Diversion Control said...

"A lot of people don't know Ritalin is like cocaine. That doesn't mean don't use it. ...It can be very dangerous and must be treated with respect."

C3CRC3CR

In the TRANS-ACTION MAGAZINE, July/August 1971, Charles Witter wrote about "DRUGGING and SCHOOLING"
"...A careful reading of Department of Health Education, and Welfare (HEW) testimony at the Gallagher hearing suggests that **200,000** children in the United States are now being given amphetamine and stimulant therapy..."

CRCRCRCR

"NEWSWEEK" - March 18, 1996
"More than **1,000,000** American children take Ritalin regularly to help them with Attention Deficit disorder, an increase of two and a half times since 1990. Do we have a miracle cure—or over-medicated kids?"

CRCRCRCR

"CHICAGO SUN-TIMES" - METRO - March 22, 1998
"With at least **10 percent of all American boys ages 6 to 14** now on stimulants for severe attention

problems, chances are that someone in your child's elementary school classroom is taking the drug Ritalin each morning before heading to school.

At least **3,500,000** American children take Ritalin and its generic counterpart, methylphenidate. We consume five times as much of the drug today than a decade ago and consume 90 percent of the worldwide market, drug enforcement officials say."

ೞೀೞೀೞೀೞೀ

Peter R. Breggin, M.D., in his book <u>Talking Back To Ritalin</u> 1998, Common Courage Press, writes...

"It's 9:00 a.m. on a school day. Do you know what your children are on? Ritalin, Dexedrine, Adderall, Desoxyn, Gradumet, Cylert, amphetamines?

Have you wondered whether your child's behavior might be helped by these drugs? Has a teacher or doctor suggested this to you? If so, you need the facts—facts that most doctors can't tell you because even doctors haven't been told the truth about the drugs that they prescribe. Did you know that:

• Ritalin doesn't correct biochemical imbalances - it causes them.
• Ritalin causes gross abnormalities in brain function.

- Labeling children ADHA and treating them with Ritalin can keep them out of the armed forces, limit their future careers, and stigmatize them for life.
- Ritalin can cause the same bad effects as amphetamine and cocaine, including behavioral disorders, growth suppression, neurological tics, agitation, addiction, and psychosis.

ଓଢ଼ଓଢ଼

"IMPACT" the CNN & TIME newsmagazine, on Special Assignment in 1997 Cable News Network, Inc. correspondent Larry LeMotte reported on...

Ritalin: The Smart Pill?

"The latest drug rage on our college campuses: a prescription pill that does help grade school children, but when abused by older students, can be deadly.

Drug of Choice

Nuevo Laredo, Mexico... Bargains for sale at the border.

At the top of his list, Ritalin the prescription drug meant to help some younger children focus better in school.

For older students today, it is the latest drug of choice for misuse -- and abuse.

College students call Ritalin the "smart pill." They swallow it as an all-night stimulant to study, or snort it as a party drug. To them, it's a harmless high, even though experts say Ritalin can be as powerful as cocaine -- and sometimes as dangerous."

೮೩೦೩೦೩೦೩

Chicago Sun-Times on November 24, 1998 reported that **Time Shows the Dark Side of Ritalin...**

"*Time* magazine (November 30, 1998) ... Already, according to *Time*, teens are trying Ritalin by purchasing them for $5 a pop, grinding them up and snorting them."

೮೩೦೩೦೩೦೩

Chicago Sun-Times, December 9, 1998, in an article "Drugging of Our Kids Creates a Ritalin Nation" writes...

"The Food and Drug Administration issued new rules 10 days ago that require drug companies to study more thoroughly the safety and effectiveness of drugs for children. Staggering though it is to believe, many drugs regularly prescribed to children have been tested only on adults. Even their labels admit as much: "Safety and effectiveness in pediatric patients have not been established." Nonetheless,

Chapter VII - Page 177

these drugs are peddled to children, while unwitting parents and society turn a blind eye to the unknown and potentially disastrous long-term effects...

...The FDA decision coincides with a report issued by the National Institutes of Health, which conceded that for the most widely medicated childhood "condition"—attention deficit disorder—"there is no current, validated diagnostic test."

This hasn't stopped prescriptions of Ritalin to children who've been given a diagnosis of Attention Deficit Hyperactivity Disorder from jumping to 75 percent in 1996, up 20 percent since 1989. At the same time, the percentage of those receiving psychotherapy dropped from 40 percent to 25 percent. Such statistics highlight the crass, bottom-line approach of most health care providers, who prefer relatively cheap drugs to costly therapy. But they also speak to our lazy culture's inclination to medicate major social problems rather than act on them.

When the government spends $16 billion a year on the drug war, and when more than half of those in jail are nonviolent drug offenders, isn't it time we connected the dots between prescription drugs and street drugs? How many more prisons do we have to build to jail offenders whom, earlier in life, we had drugged with abandon?"

ଓଷଓଷଓଷ

A study by Zito, et al., published in the *Journal of the American Medical Association*, February 2000, raises disturbing questions about whether its safe to prescribe psychotropic drugs to toddlers. The study examined trends between 1991 and 1995. Ritalin use doubled or tripled depending on the group. Use of anti-depressants increased by 30%. They also reported that Ritalin has not been studied on children under age 4 and the label warns against its use in children under the age of 6...

"The possibility of adverse effects on the developing brain cannot be ruled out... And that earlier starts on medicine mean that children will likely take the drug for longer periods. The long term consequences should be studied."

Zito also questioned whether its possible to make an accurate diagnosis of depression or ADHD in toddlers.

ଓଷଓଷଓଷ

Bias

Bias - "A particular tendency or inclination, especially one that prevents impartial consideration of a question"
Webster's College Dictionary

The American Academy of Pediatrics in 1971went public with "**AAP Releases TV Public Service Announcement On Hyperactive Child**".

"Continuing to expand its public education program the American Academy of Pediatrics has released its fifth television public service announcement to 500 TV stations across the nation. The announcement on the hyperkinetic child is the fourth TV spot developed this year. One spot was released in 1970.

The announcement has been completely financed by CIBA Pharmaceutical Company, Summit, N.J...."

ଔଔଔଔ

USA Today on November 16, 1995, reports "Ritalin Maker's Ties to Advocates Probed" reports...

"Government officials are questioning the relationship between the manufacturers of the drug Ritalin, widely used to treat children with attention deficit disorders, and a high-profile parent advocacy group.

After a year-long investigation, the United Nations and the U.S. Drug Enforcement Administration say financial ties between the company, Ciba-Geigy, and Children and Adults with Attention Deficit Disorders may be putting profit margins ahead of child safety.

The drug manufacturer admits to funding a portion of CHADD's $2 million budget. The DEA found nearly $1 million in funding, growing from $100,000 in 1991 to $398,000 in 1994.

According to October DEA documents, the agency fears the financial relationship is "not well-known by the public, including CHADD members that have relied upon CHADD for guidance."

The International Narcotics Control Board, the DEA reports, is concerned about CHADD's recent lobbying efforts to reclassify Ritalin. At present, the stimulant is subject to strict prescription guidelines, in the same category as amphetamines and morphine. Reclassification would make it cheaper and more accessible.

 C3C3C3C3

Side Effects

"IMPACT" the CNN Interactive & TIME newsmagazine, on Special Assignment, November 9, 1998, CNN.com, reported on...

Group Issues Guidelines for Monitoring Ritalin in Children

"Reports of sudden death in children and teenagers treated with psychotropic drugs such as Ritalin have prompted the American Heart

Association to issue guidelines for proper drug
monitoring.

Drugs like the popular Ritalin and other psycho-
stimulant medications, which are often used to treat
children or adolescents with attention deficit
hyperactivity disorder or ADHA, have been
associated with increased cardiovascular risks.

Doctors say while some psychotropic medications
may cause sudden death, in general, Ritalin taken
alone is very safe.

According to guidelines, before a child starts
treatment, careful medical and family histories
should be obtained to screen for heart palpitations,
heart conduction problems or fainting spells. If
there are any such concerns, the child should be
referred to a cardiologist before starting medication."

છ૪ઇ૪છ૪ઇ૪

**Physician's Desk Reference entry for
RITALIN (NOVARTIS PHARMACEUTICALS)**

"CONTRAINDICATIONS: Marked anxiety, tension,
and agitation are contraindications to Ritalin, since
the drug may aggravate these symptoms. Ritalin is
contraindicated also in patients known to be
hypersensitive to the drug, in patients with

glaucoma, and in patients with motor tics or with a family history or diagnosis of Tourette's syndrome.

WARNINGS: Ritalin should not be used in children under six years, since safety and efficacy in this age group have not been established. Sufficient data on safety and efficacy of long-term use of Ritalin in children are not yet available. Although a causal relationship has not been established, suppression of growth (i.e., weight gain, and/or height) has been reported with the long-term use of stimulants in children. Therefore, patients requiring long-term therapy should be carefully monitored.

DRUG DEPENDENCE: Ritalin should be given cautiously to emotionally unstable patients, such as those with a history of drug dependence or alcoholism, because such patients may increase dosage on their own initiative. Chronically abusive use can lead to marked tolerance and psychic dependence with varying degrees of abnormal behavior. Frank psychotic episodes can occur, especially with parenteral abuse. Careful supervision is required during drug withdrawal, since severe depression as well as the effects of chronic over activity can be unmasked. Long-term follow-up may be required because of the patient's basic personality disturbances.

ADVERSE REACTIONS: Nervousness and insomnia are the most common adverse reactions but are usually controlled by reducing dosage and omitting the drug in the afternoon or evening. Other reactions include hypersensitivity (including skin rash, urticaria, fever, arthralgia, exfoliative dermatitis, erythema multiforme with histopathological findings of necrotizing vasculitis, and thrombocytopenic purpura); anorexia; nausea; dizziness; palpitations; headache; dyskinesia; drowsiness; blood pressure and pulse changes, both up and down; tachycardia; angina; cardiac arrhythmia; abdominal pain; weight loss during prolonged therapy. There have been rare reports of Tourette's syndrome. Toxic psychosis has been reported. Although a definite causal relationship has not been established, the following have been reported in patients taking this drug: instances of abnormal liver function, ranging from transaminase elevation to hepatic coma; isolated cases of cerebral arteritis and/or occlusion; leukopenia and/or anemia; transient depressed mood; a few instances of scalp hair loss. Very rare reports of neuroleptic malignant syndrome (NMS) have been received, and, in most of these, patients were concurrently receiving therapies associated with NMS. In a single report, a ten year old boy who had been taking methylphenidate for approximately 18 months experienced an NMS-like event within 45 minutes of ingesting his first dose of venlaxafine. It is uncertain whether this case represented a drug-drug interaction, a response to either drug alone, or some other cause. In children, loss of appetite, abdominal pain, weight loss during prolonged therapy, insomnia, and tachycardia may occur more frequently; however, any of the other adverse reactions listed above may also occur.

CBCRCBCR

Next Up Prozac

"Time Magazine" on November 30, 1998 - page 94, in an article by Jeffrey Kluger wrote...

"When you're 10 years old, you shouldn't have much to be depressed about—or so an adult might think. But just as more and more children are taking Ritalin to calm their hyperactivity storms, a growing number of kids are turning to Prozac and other antidepressants to treat their blues...

...Meanwhile, Prozac's manufacturer, Eli Lilly is conducting clinical studies in the under-18 age group, and may have just the product for this booming new market: liquid Prozac flavored a tasty peppermint."

CBCRCBCR

Ritalin

REFERENCES

Block, Dr. Mary Ann , <u>No More Ritalin : Treating ADHD Without Drugs</u>, 1997, Mass Market Paperback.

Breggin, M.D., Peter Roger, <u>Talking Back to Ritalin : What Doctors Aren't Telling You About Stimulants for Children</u>, 1998, Common Courage Press

Diller, M.D., Lawrence H., <u>Running on Ritalin : A Physician Reflects on Children, Society, and Performance in a Pill</u>, September 1, 1998. Bantam Doubleday Dell Pub.

Newsweek magazine, March 18, 1996

Szasz, M.D., Thomas S., <u>The Manufacture of Madness : A Comparative Study of the Inquisition and the Mental Health Movement,</u> Reprint edition (June 1997), Syracuse Univ Pr.

Time magazine, November 30, 1998

www.homefirst.com

Chapter VIII

The Birth Control "Pill"
Unavoidably Dangerous

"Choose Life"

Deuteronomy 30:19

No other drug in the Physician's Desk Reference has as long a description of side effects as the birth control "PILL." Breast cancer, cardiovascular disease, blood clots, liver tumors, high blood pressure, infertility, sterility, and abortion are some of the more serious problems associated with the "PILL." In fact, the new third generation "PILL" seems to be more dangerous than the previous ones. This is not surprising. The late Dr. Mendelsohn said, "Doctors don't let go of one medication until they find a more dangerous one to replace it." The dangers of the "PILL" are well documented. Doctors believe that no woman should be deprived of her "PILL" (a form of chemical steroids) so they prescribe the "PILL" for a list of completely contra-indicated medical conditions such as: irregular periods, scanty periods, no periods, ovarian cysts and even acne. When asked about the side effects of the "PILL" most doctors will tell you, *"trust me, it's safer than being pregnant."* This thinking reflects most doctor's views that pregnancy is a disease for which the "PILL" is the cure. As a

blessed and proud father of six children and a doubly
blessed grandfather of six grandchildren, I am proud that
my wife, daughters, and daughter-in-law have never been on
the "PILL". If you are a teenager don't take the "PILL"! If you
are thinking about ever having children, don't take the
"PILL"!! If you're not thinking of having children, don't take
the "PILL"!!! The "PILL" is unavoidably dangerous. As a
medical student in 1971, I met Dr. Herbert Ratner. This
distinguished physician and mentor became one of the most
inspiring people in my life. Not only did Dr. Ratner teach
my wife, Karen, and I the importance of children and family,
he also informed us of the medical risks and hazards of the
"PILL."

ଔଔଔଔ

It is with great pleasure that I present an editorial
written by the late Dr. Herbert Ratner;

<u>The Medical Hazards of the Birth Control Pill</u>
"To withdraw a drug once on the market is
considerably more difficult than to get a drug on the
market. FDA originally approved The Pill (Enovid) as
safe for marketing on the basis of studies on only
132 women who had taken The Pill consecutively for
12 or more months. (Morton Mintz, *By Prescription
Only*, Houghton Mifflin Co, Boston, 1967, p. 271.)
Since The Pill has been on the market, the number
of deaths reported in association with The Pill has

far exceeded this number. In fact, it is safe to say that The Pill is the most dangerous drug ever introduced for use by the healthy in respect to lethality and major complications.

To admit mistakes is not characteristic of the American scene. Governmental agencies are no exceptions. In addition, the pressures and manipulations by drug firms—and the people they subsidize—to prevent a drug from being removed from the market can be extraordinary.

This is especially true of The Pill. Everyone prefers to believe that The Pill is safe.

The net result of propaganda, which led to pronouncements of Pill safety out of so-called humanitarian considerations, was that the real users of The Pill, the middle and upper classes of the U.S., were seduced away from well established and safe means of birth control.

Perhaps the most fallacious argument in defense of The Pill is that it prevents the hazards of pregnancy. How a Pill which places the woman in a continuous state of false pregnancy, which in turn reproduces the illnesses of occasional pregnancies, can be considered an advantage is beyond scientific comprehension. The English, in an attempt to water down their finding of 3 deaths per 100,000 women from thromboembolism by alleging that The Pill prevents 12 deaths per 100,000 from pregnancy, ignore two essential facts. The first is that the alternative to The Pill is not pregnancy, but other and safer means of conception control. The second is that prior poor health contributes to most of the deaths in pregnancy. Contrasting the death rate of healthy women on The Pill to healthy pregnant women results in an entirely different comparison.

In pregnancy, the vascular system of the body adjusts to accommodate a rapidly enlarging uterus. In false or Pill induced pseudopregnancy, the pelvic vascular system increases the blood supply, but there is no enlarging uterus to utilize the increase. This results in extensive pelvic venous congestion, a condition which causes distress to surgeons. Such unnatural congestion introduces a whole series of factors predisposing to thrombosis and embolic phenomena.

The second example relates to the hypercoaguable state of pregnancy. This state was described prior to the introduction of The Pill. (B. Alexander, M.D., et al, Increased Clotting Factors in Pregnancy, New England Journal of Medicine 256:10931097, Nov. 30, 1961.) "This (state) provides a means whereby rapid clotting may take place at the site of placental separation." (Louise L. Phillips, Ch. 12, "Modifications of the Coagulation Mechanism During

Pregnancy," in Modern Trends in Human Reproductive Physiology, Ed. H. M. Carey, Butterworths, 1963.) The Pill duplicates the hypercoaguable state. Because it serves no function in false pregnancy, its only contribution is to make the "patient potentially more susceptible to intravascular thrombosis." (Ibid,) The Pill introduces the risk without compensatory advantage.

The third example relates to the well known protection that pregnancy or embryonic tissue confer against certain induced cancers. In the absence of fetal tissue this protection is not conferred. We cannot assume that using The Pill contraceptively, confers this fetal-maternal relationship to human beings.

It would seem that if we had any respect for nature's economics, subtleties and the ordering of health, and any humility with respect to our multiple ignorances of the fetal-maternal relationship, we would more readily recognize that a state of false pregnancy is pathologic.

The first committee appointed to study the question of thromboembolism, in relation to The Pill, was sponsored by the manufacturers of Enovid, not the government, and conducted by the American Medical Association. (Proceedings of a Conference: Thromboembolic Phenomena in Women, Sept. 10,

1962, Chicago) The latter has a well known bias in favor of the pharmaceutical industry. Within several hours of convening this meeting, before participants had an adequate opportunity to study and discuss the data presented at the meeting, the Chairman called for a vote that would, in effect, be a whitewash of The Pill.

He commented, ". . . so far there has not been a single shred of evidence that has been presented in any of these figures to suggest that it contributes to a greater incidence of this disease. . . Will everyone agree with that?" The Chairman ultimately got the vote he requested. That it was not unanimous is a tribute to Stanford Wessler, M.D. a leading authority on thrombosis, who with courage and perspicacity, was the single dissenting voice.

If, for reasons of its own, the FDA feels it cannot remove The Pill from the market on the same basis as other drugs, we would urge the FDA to appoint another committee. If the safety of the public is paramount, such a committee should be sympathetic to a long established principle of medicine - *Above All Do No Harm!*

CSCRCSCR

Physician's Desk Reference 2000 - Excerpt from patient package insert

The serious side effects of the pill occur very infrequently, especially if you are in good health and are young. However, you should know that the following medical conditions have been associated with or made worse by the pill:

1. Blood clots in the legs (thrombophlebitis), lungs (pulmonary embolism), stoppage or rupture of a blood vessel in the brain (stroke), blockage of blood vessels in the heart (heart attack or angina pectoris) or other organs of the body.

2. Liver tumors, which may rupture and cause severe bleeding. A possible but not definite association has been found with the pill and liver cancer. However, liver cancers are extremely rare. The chance of developing liver cancer from using the pill is thus even rarer.

3. High blood pressure, although blood pressure usually returns to normal when the pill is stopped.

ᏨᏋᏨᏋ

Third generation oral contraception and venous thromboembolism

In April 1997 the *British Medical Journal* reported...

"The published evidence confirms the Committee on Safety of Medicine's concerns

All studies indicated a statistically significant doubling of the adjusted odds ratios for venous thromboembolism in patients taking third rather than second generation oral contraceptive pills. These results are consistent with those from the transnational study published in this issue of the *British Medical Journal.* The increased risk cannot be explained by known or expected bias or confounding.

The first law of epidemiology is that if a causal effect is large enough, it will show up despite all the problems of performing, analyzing, and interpreting observational studies on real people.

The doubling of risk of venous thromboembolism in users of third generation pills is important when the baseline risk in users of the pill is already three times greater than in non-users. Some studies have reported a relative risk of venous thrombo-embolism of about nine for users of third generation pills compared to women using non-hormonal contraception."

ದ⊰ಞ⊰

Oral Contraceptives and Risk for
Breast Cancer in Young Woman

The following is text of a press release from the British National Cancer Institute Press Office. The research was reported in the Journal of the National Cancer Institute.

"A new study headed by scientists at the National Cancer Institute (NCI) adds to the evidence that oral contraceptives increase the risk of breast cancer in women under age 35. - *CancerNet News UK* June 6, 1995

'While the findings are reason for caution, breast cancer is uncommon in this age group, and the pill appears to be responsible for only a minority of breast cancers in young women,' said NCI's Louise A. Brinton, Ph.D., lead researcher of the study."

෩෫෩෫

Sterility & INFERTILITY

Progress in Contraception Control: The Sequential Regimen. Physicians' Conference, San Francisco, April 4, 1965. Mead Johnson & Co., 1965.

". . . our multiparous patients . . . want to know how long it will be after they discontinue the tablets before they can expect to conceive... We have six patients who as yet have not become pregnant. They have been trying to conceive from two months up to thirty months. Because all have previously had children, we felt there must be some reason for the delay in conceiving." - *A. L. Banks, M.D. (University of Washington)*

"I now have eight patients who are experiencing amenorrhea after discontinuing the combined contraceptive regimen . . . hoping to get pregnant. . ." - *Robert H. Hall, M.D. (University of Utah)*

"Dr. Hall, you strike a very important chord in this discussion. I think Dr. Banks made reference to this point. All of us have encountered amenorrheic episodes following termination of the combined form of therapy." - *Robert B. Greenblatt, M.D. (Medical College of Georgia)*

ೞೞೞೞ

Amenorrhea After Treatment With Oral Contraceptives. R. P. Shearman M.D. (University of Sydney. Australia).

"In a period of 6 months, 9 women with secondary amenorrhea of at least 12 months duration, gave a history of onset after stopping The Pill." - *Lancet 2:1110-1111, Nov. 19, 1966.*

*Syndrome of Anovulation Following Oral Contraceptives.
O. I. Dodek, Jr., M.D. et al (Washington, D.C. Hospital
Center).*

"The anovulation syndrome is found in patients
who have had amenorrhea or evidence of anovulation
for three or more months after discontinuance of
The Pill. Prolonged dysfunction of hypothalamic
centers concerned with cyclic gonadotropin release is
probably the cause." - *Am. J. Ob. and Gyn. 98 :1065-
1070, 1967.*

*Clomiphene Citrate for Improvement of Ovarian Function
Georgeanna Seegar Jones, M.D. and Maria D. de Moraes-
Ruehsen, M.D. (Johns Hopkins University).*

"There were four women with longstanding
amenorrhea (sterility) following oral contraception
therapy." - *Am. J. Ob. & Gyn. 99:814-828, Nov. 15,
1967.*

*Irregular Menses, Amenorrhea and Infertility Following
Synthetic Progestational Agents. M. James Whitelaw, M.D. et
al.*

"During the past year we have had occasion to see
24 patients with normal menstrual cycles, but who,
following the use of synthetic progestational agents
(The Pill), had one or more of the following
conditions as their chief complaint: irregular

menses, amenorrhea, and infertility."
Communication with other clinics indicates that
there are hundreds of such cases that are
unreported. "Let's Be Honest About The Pill" and
inform nulliparous women, and those with only one
living child of the possibility of being relatively
infertile for undeterminate periods of time following
discontinuation of oral contraceptives. " - *JAMA
195:780-782, Feb. 28,1966.*

*Should Nullipara and Infertility Patients be Given Oral
Contraceptives? M. James Whitelaw, M.D. (Chief of Infertility
Clinic, Santa Clara County Medical Center).*

"Nullipara and infertility patients should not be
given The Pill." - *New England Obstetrical and
Gynecological Society, 39th Annual Meeting, Nov. 1,
1967.*

ඏණඏණ

National Center for Health Statistics , 1988

In 1988 a panel assembled by the Congressional Office
of Technology Assessment presented the following statistics
to the U.S. Congress. Twenty five percent of couples in their
thirties are infertile, even though only 1% of teenagers are
infertile.

ඏණඏණ

Wall Street Journal, 1993

Self-made Swiss billionaire, Fabio Bertarelli, whose company Serono Laboratories, manufactures 70 percent of the world's gonadotrophic hormones to treat infertility (including Pergonal and Metrodin), confirms this. In 1993 Bertarelli told the *Wall Street Journal,* "Our usual customers are women over 30 who have been taking birth-control pills since they were teenagers or in their early 20s."

ଔଓଔଓ

The Couples' Guide to Infertility, 1995

In the 1995 revised edition, Dr. Gary S. Berger and his associates again confirm the observations of Maggie Humm and Fabio Bertareli. "Long-term pill users may not menstruate or ovulate after they stop using the pill. This condition, known as post-pill amenorrhea, occurs because the pill disrupts the natural rhythmic flow of hormones from the hypothalamus to the pituitary to the ovaries. This may post a special problem for older women who have been on the pill for many years because their ovaries may have become resistant to resuming ovulation."

ଔଓଔଓ

Cardiovascular Impact

Dr. Meir J. Stampfer in the *New England Journal of Medicine*, November 24, 1988 reported on the cardiovascular impacts of the birth control pill...

"The most dangerous and well-documented side effects commonly associated with the Pill are heart attacks and strokes. The eight-year Nurse's Health Study at Harvard Medical School found that Pill users are 250 percent as likely to have heart attacks and strokes than those who don't use the Pill, probably because the Pill excessively increases blood clotting ability.

However, one of the major findings of the study was that women who get off the Pill have rates of cardiovascular disease equal to that of the general population after a period of one year.

This study was based on an eight-year followup of 119,061 female nurses, ranging in age from 30 to 55 in 1980. 7,074 were current pill users and 49,269 were previous users. Overall, there was 380 heart attacks, 205 strokes, and 230 cardiovascular deaths among pill users."

 C3C3C3C3

Unavoidably Unsafe

Thomas P. Monaghan, Co-Chairman, Free Speech Advocates wrote an article "Unavoidably Unsafe" in *Fidelity* Magazine, October 1987, pages 14 and 15...

"According to United States Federal Courts, the birth control pill has been classified as 'unavoidably unsafe.' This means that, implicit in a woman's consent to use the pill, even if she is not entirely informed of its dangers, is an acknowledgment of physical risk."

ଓଊଓଊ

Disturbing Information on the Pill

Dr. Ojvind Lidepaard, et al., Hvidovre University Clinic of Copenhagen, reporting in the *British Medical Journal* (April 1993 cited *Europe Today* No. 23, May 3, 1993) revealed that in a study of 2400 women aged 15 to 44, who were using the Birth control Pill, 800 suffered some degree of cerebral thrombosis. although not all of the blood clots led to stroke.

ଓଊଓଊ

The "Pill" as Abortifacient

*Whoever causes the loss of a single soul is as
though he caused the loss of a world entire, and
whoever saves one is as though he saved a
universe*

Talmud, Sanhedrin

In addition to all the serious side effects of the Pill (**i.e.
blood clots, stroke, high blood pressure, breast cancer,
etc. to name just a few**), the Pill can cause abortions.

To label the Pill only as a contraceptive is misleading.
Webster's Unabridged Dictionary defines contraception as
"artificial prevention of the fertilization of the human ovum,
often called birth control." Abortion is defined by Webster's
Unabridged Dictionary as "the act of producing young before
the natural time." By not allowing the baby to implant in the
mother's uterus, one of the modes of action of the Pill is not
contraception, but abortion. Even while taking the pill a
pregnancy can still occur, but implantation of the baby into
the uterus cannot happen. The difference between
contraception and abortion is not subtle. It is the difference
between preventing a conception and causing an abortion.
There is no distinction between one second of life, one year

of life, ten years of life, etc. If we accept the principle that life begins at conception, then there is no difference if we end life (with usage of the Pill) by chemical abortion, at six days after conception or ten weeks after conception by surgical abortion. Abortion is abortion; different methods don't change the fact that a life has been ended.

Users of the "old" high-dosage birth control pills experienced relatively severe side effects. However, many of these pills were generally considered non-abortifacient in their two-fold ("biphasic") modes of action. The pills would thicken cervical mucus and inhibit ovulation, but they would generally *not* inhibit implantation of the blastocyst (the five-day old, 256-cell developing human being) in the uterine lining.

However, the new low-dosage pills are "triphasic." They have three modes of action; they thicken cervical mucus, inhibit ovulation, *and* block implantation. Therefore, the "new" Pills are *all* abortifacient in nature. These actions explain why the minipill works, as it generally does not suppress ovulation.

Many women, including those who are pro-life, who would never even *consider* a surgical abortion now use low-dose birth control pills that may cause them to abort on an average of once or twice every year. A large number of pro-life women use these pills, and most do not know the Pill has this mode of action.

Birth Control Pill

The pharmaceutical manufacturers of the Pill have outlined at least three modes of action. First, the Pill prevents ovulation, second, the Pill decreases sperm conductivity and third, the Pill alters the lining of the uterus, not allowing the baby to implant into the uterine wall. It is this third method that actually causes the abortion. Randy Alcorn, in his outstanding treatise, "Does the birth control pill cause abortion?" brings much scientific evidence to explain how the Pill causes abortions. This issue of abortion places a discussion about the use of the Pill in a different light. Even if the Pill had no other side effects, from a pro-life perspective alone, it would not be acceptable.

One must remember that not taking the Pill does not necessarily mean becoming pregnant and having a baby. **We do have other choices,** i.e. other safer means of birth control, such as condoms, diaphragms, natural family planning, and the choice of abstinence. Doctors and pharmaceutical companies have led us to believe that without the pill every woman would become pregnant with each act of intercourse. This is truly a false impression that has no scientific basis. The window of opportunity for fertility is only about three days per month. The sad reality is that over 30% of women have infertility problems.

Why have we not been told about this effect of the Pill which causes abortions? I believe it is the same forces in our society which promote promiscuity, sex outside of marriage, and in general unhealthy lifestyles which have suppressed this information. At present there are over 14 million women in the United States on the Pill. This amounts to a multi-billion dollar industry. This industry preys on the public's perception that promiscuity is unavoidable. All we have to do is look to our so-called "role models" (i.e. popular magazines, youth oriented television programs, sports and our political leaders) to see lifestyles that endorse promiscuity and sexual unfaithfulness. A recent issue of "Time" magazine had the headline "Are Parents Actually Necessary?" Are we living the precepts outlined in Huxley's novel *Brave New World*? Has yesterday's fiction become today's reality? Let us strive in every aspect of our life to choose life over death. As such let us reject the Pill.

ೞೞೞೞ

Edited excerpts from Randy Alcorn's "Does the Birth Control Pill Cause Abortions?" as it appears on the Internet.

"Contraceptives" That Aren't Contraceptives

Contraceptives are chemicals or devices that prevent conception. A birth control method that kills an already conceived person is not a contraceptive, it is an abortifacient... Pro-life advocates have long opposed the use of Intra-Uterine Devices (IUDs), because they do not prevent conception, but keep the already conceived child from implanting in his mother's womb. Likewise, we oppose RU-486, the anti-progesterone abortion pill. RU-486 is a human pesticide, causing a mother's womb to become hostile to her own child, resulting in an induced miscarriage. Depo-Provera is an anti-progesterone injected every three months. It sometimes suppresses ovulation, but also thins the lining of the uterus, preventing implantation. Norplant is another anti-progesterone drug enclosed in five or six flexible closed capsules or rods, which are surgically implanted beneath the skin. It often suppresses ovulation, but sometimes ovulation occurs, and when it does an irritation to the uterine wall often prevents implantation. The Emergency Contraceptive Pill (ECP) also known as the "Morning After Pill" does not prevent pregnancy, but keeps a fertilized egg from implanting in the uterus. All of these birth control methods either sometimes or often alter the mother's womb in a way that causes it to reject the human life which God designed it to nourish and sustain... These birth control methods are often referred to as "contraceptives," but they are not exclusively contraceptives. That is, they do not always prevent conception, but sometimes or often result in the death of already conceived human beings... The FDA-required research information on the birth control pills Ortho-Cyclen and Ortho

Tri-Cyclen also state that they cause "changes in . . . the endometrium (which reduce the likelihood of implantation)." (The PDR, 1995, page 1782). Notice that these changes in the endometrium, and their reduction in the likelihood of implantation, are not stated by the manufacturer as speculative or theoretical effects, but as actual ones... Similarly, Syntex, another major Pill manufacturer, says this in Physician's Desk Reference (1995, page 2461) under the "Clinical Pharmacology" of the six pills it produces (two types of Brevicon and four of Norinyl): Although the primary mechanism of this action is inhibition of ovulation, other alterations include changes in the cervical mucus (which increase the difficulty of sperm entry into the uterus), and the endometrium (which may reduce the likelihood of implantation). Wyeth, on page 2685 of The PDR, 1995, says something very similar of its combination Pills, including Lo/Ovral and Ovral: "other alterations include changes in the cervical mucus . . . and changes in the endometrium which reduce the likelihood of implantation." Wyeth makes virtually identical statements about its birth control pills Nordette (The PDR, 1995, page 2693) and Triphasil (page 2743). The medical textbook Williams Obstetrics (Cunningham, et al, Stamford, CT: Appleton & Lange, 1993, page 1323) states, "Similar

Chapter VIII - Page 207

to estrogens, progestins produce an endometrium that is unfavorable to blastocyst implantation." Drug Facts and Comparisons says this about birth control pills in its 1996 edition: Combination OCs inhibit ovulation by suppressing the gonadotropins, follicle-stimulating hormone (FSH) and lutenizing hormone (LH). Additionally, alterations in the genital tract, including cervical mucus (which inhibits sperm penetration) and the endometrium (which reduces the likelihood of implantation), may contribute to contraceptive effectiveness.   "The Pill: How does it work? Is it safe?" (The Couple to Couple League, PO Box 111184, Cincinnati, OH, 45211) states on page 4: "When the Pill fails to prevent ovulation, the other mechanisms come into play. Thickened cervical mucus may make it more difficult for the sperm to reach the egg: however, if the egg is fertilized, a new life is created. The hormones slow the transfer of the new life through the fallopian tube, and the embryo may become too old to be viable when it does enter the uterus.   If the embryo is still viable when it reaches the uterus, underdevelopment of the uterine lining caused by the Pill prevents implantation. The embryo dies and the remains are passed along in the next bleeding episode which, incidentally, is not a true menstruation, even though it is usually perceived as such."

In her article Abortifacient Drugs and Devices:
Medical and Moral Dilemmas (Linacre Quarterly,
August 1990, page 55), Dr. Kristine Severyn states,
The third effect of combined oral contraceptives is to
alter the endometrium in such a way that
implantation of the fertilized egg (new life) is made
more difficult, if not impossible. In effect, the
endometrium becomes atrophic and unable to
support implantation of the fertilized egg. . . . the
alteration of the endometrium, making it hostile to
implantation by the fertilized egg, provides a backup
abortifacient method to prevent pregnancy.
Pro-abortionists know it: Why don't we?   If most
pro-lifers have been slow to catch on to this
established medical knowledge... In his brochure
"How the Pill and the IUD Work: Gambling with Life"
(American Life League, P.O. Box 1350, Stafford, VA
22555), Dr. David Sterns asks: Just how often does
the pill have to rely on this abortive 'backup'
mechanism? No one can tell you with certainty.
Perhaps it is as seldom as 1 to 2% of the time, but
perhaps it is as frequently as 50% of the time. Does
it matter? The clear conclusion is that it is
impossible for any woman on the pill in any given
month to know exactly which mechanism is in effect.
In other words, the pill always carries with it the
potential to act as an abortifacient. Even when the

information leaks out, so many pro-life advocates --
including pastors and parachurch leaders -- have
used and recommended the Pill, that we have a
natural resistance to raising this issue or looking
into it seriously when others raise it. This is likely
why so few individuals or organizations have
researched or drawn attention to this subject.

M.E. Comments:

*I recommend that you read the complete version of Alcorn's
outstanding treatise on "Does the Birth Control Pill Cause
Abortions?". It is imperative that every person who believes
that life begins at conception understands that the birth
control pill is also an abortifacient.*

෬෪෬෪෬෪෬෪

REFERENCES

Berger, Dr. Gary S., The Couples' Guide to Infertility, 1995.

Couple to Couple League's website is http://www.ccli.org

Epstein, et al., The Breast Cancer Prevention Program, "Chapter 3, The Pill: Assessing Your Risks," Macmillan, U.S.A.

http://www.epm.org/bcpill1.htm - for entire article by Randy Alcorn - "Does the Birth Control Pill Cause Abortions?" 2nd edition, Revised March 1998, also available through a link on the Homefirst® web site.

http://www.homefirst.com (The Homefirst® WEB page containing extensive links to research on the "Pill", as well as many related topics).

Mintz, Morton, The Pill An Alarming Report, (*Washington Post)* 1969.

Ratner, Herbert, M.D., "The Medical Hazards of the Birth Control Pill," Child and Family, 1970.

Seaman, Barbara, The Doctor's Case Against the Pill, 1995 (original publication 1969), Hunter House.

Chapter IX

Synthetic Hormone Replacement Therapy
Unavoidably Dangerous

Did God make American women deficient in estrogen and progesterone? Does every American woman need synthetic chemical estrogen or progesterone chemicals when they reach menopause? Do synthetic hormones protect women from heart disease and osteoporosis? Is a synthetic hormone, which is structurally different, better than a natural hormone? Is every phase of our lives a condition that must be treated with chemical drugs?

WHAT ARE SYNTHETIC HORMONES ??

The pharmaceutical companies that compound synthetic hormones are brilliant. They have ingeniously developed synthetic estrogen and progesterone compounds which, in many ways, mimic the body's own estrogen and progesterone. In order to patent their designer estrogen and progestin products, they must alter the natural chemical structure. These altered synthetic chemicals have been linked to many serious side-effects (a partial listing from the PDR [Physicians Desk Reference] includes high blood pressure, blood clots in the lung, brain, headaches, changes in libido, fatigue, hirsutism, hemorrhagic eruptions, coagulation problems). Hormones are messengers which instruct different cells in our body to perform various tasks. By taking exogenous (introduced from or produced outside the human body) hormones we are able to give the body instructions that the body would not normally give itself. By taking synthetic estrogen and synthetic progesterone during one's reproductive life, messages are sent telling the body not to ovulate or not to let the fertilized egg implant into the uterus. Use of these hormones can lessen or eliminate pre-menopausal and menopausal symptoms. The question is what price are we paying for these alleged benefits? Are there other, safer means available?

THE PRICE OF SYNTHETIC HORMONES

Increased risk for blood clots, stroke, and cancer are just a part of the price that we are paying for ingesting synthetic hormones. But why? The hormone messengers that our body produces are very specific. Even a small alteration in the hormone's structure can bring about a completely different message. The difference in the

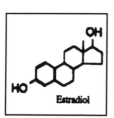

Figure 1
Estradiol - one
of the body's
natural
estrogens.

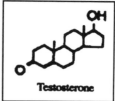

Figure 2
Natural
testosterone.

Chapter IX - Page 214

structure between estradiol (one of the body's natural estrogens - see Figure 1) and testosterone (see Figure 2), is seemingly very little. The difference is the HO attachment to estradiol vs. the O attachment to testosterone on the bottom of the hormone molecule. Yet, we know that the production of estradiol by the body will cause feminization and the production of testosterone will cause masculinization.

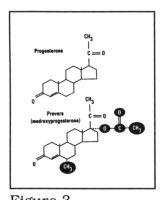

Figure 3

Note the similarity between natural progesterone and Provera (one of the synthetic progestins).

The synthetic hormones sold by the drug companies (see Fig. 3) are structurally similar to those produced by the body and will produce estrogenic and testosterone effects.

However, they are not the same. The synthetic hormones are capable of producing other effects as mentioned above. The structural alteration is necessary because these synthetic compounds, if not structurally altered, would not exert their effect in a "pill" form. They would be broken down by the body or the effect would be too short lived to be effective. Natural estrogen and natural progesterone can be produced in cream forms which can be readily absorbed; however, they cannot be patented.

Synthetic Hormone Replacement Therapy

We have 50 years of history with the synthetic estrogen-like compound Diethylstilbesterol or DES during which time DES was dispensed to over 5,000,000 women. In the 1950's doctors prescribed for pregnant women the synthetic estrogen-like drug, DES, which was supposed to prevent miscarriages. Leading researchers and gynecologists hailed the man-made estrogen DES, as a wonder drug with a host of potential uses. Almost immediately, researchers began prescribing DES for women who were experiencing problems during pregnancy, in the belief that insufficient estrogen levels caused miscarriage and premature births. This would prove to be a massive human experiment.

In the decades that followed, doctors not only prescribed DES to prevent miscarriages, they began to recommend it also for untroubled pregnancies, as if it were a vitamin that could improve on nature.

In 1971, a rare vaginal cancer began being diagnosed in young women. This was linked to a drug their mothers had taken during pregnancy, the synthetic estrogen DES. Until DES, most scientists believed that the placenta acted as a barrier letting good substances in and keeping bad ones out. They believed that drugs were safely administered during pregnancy unless it caused immediate problems or obvious birth defects. The most painful aspect of the DES tragedy is that the drug did not even prevent miscarriages.

Those who took DES did not have fewer miscarriages, fewer premature babies, or fewer infant deaths. The drug,

DES, not only did not prevent miscarriages, but, increased the risk of malformation and cancer of the urogenital tract (vagina, cervix, ovaries, testes) in the children born to these women.

This tragic and unintended experiment demonstrated that chemicals could cross the placenta, disrupt the development of the baby, and have serious effects that might not be evident until decades later.

The DES experience offered another critical lesson as well, that is relevant not just to those exposed to DES, but to all of us. The developmental effects of DES made it clear that the human body could mistake a man made chemical (i.e. birth control pill, hormone replacement therapy) for a (nature made) hormone. DES was taken off the market and labeled as a cancer producing drug. Since then we have learned that all synthetic estrogen-like drugs (oral contraceptives, Premarin, Tamoxifin, Provera, Prempro, etc.) can cause cancer. There has been a dramatic rise in estrogen sensitive breast cancer. In fact, the majority of breast cancers in young women, are estrogen sensitive caused by the greater exposure to estrogen, and synthetic estrogen-like compounds.

Dr. Samuel Epstein's outstanding book, <u>The Breast Cancer Prevention Program,</u> outlines the role that synthetic estrogens play in causing breast cancer.

The lessons to be learned from these fiascos are:

    1) Drug companies sell drugs.

2) Doctors prescribe (push) drugs.

3) Doctors are influenced by drug companies and their own prejudices, not by scientific studies.

4) Doctors believe that nature made a mistake by allowing women to get pregnant.

5) Doctors believe that nature made a mistake by decreasing a woman's estrogen level, forcing them to go through menopause.

6) Doctors believe that most of life is a struggle against disease.

As prudent consumers we must courteously listen to our doctors. We must then question every one of their recommendations. Only then, after weighing the scientific evidence, should we proceed with any treatment plan. We must remind the doctors of the oath of Hippocrates that they took, "Primum Non Nocere" - Above All Do No Harm. We must attempt to improve our life style with the following methods:

1) Start by having your baby at home (avoiding hospital drugs and high cesarean section rates).

2) Breast feed your baby.

3) Avoid the birth control pill and hormone replacement therapy (synthetic altered estrogens and progesterones).

4) Question vaccinations

5) Question antibiotics

6) Avoid ingesting meat from animals that have been fed estrogen supplements and/or growth hormones.

7) Avoid milk from cows that have been injected with bovine growth hormone.

Nothing in life is a guarantee. Even if you follow all of the above principles, problems may still occur. However, statistically, you will lower your probability of problems. It is a scary thought that many of the diseases we will face in the 21st century will be caused by man, not nature produced.

Bottle feeding, vaccinations, synthetic hormones, pesticides (such as DDT, dioxin, PCBs and PVCs) are just some of the factors which have been linked to the rise in cancer and auto immune diseases (Multiple Sclerosis, Hodgkins, Fibromyalgia, Chronic Fatigue Syndrome, etc.).

We are drowning in a sea of synthetic estrogens. Not only do our doctors use synthetic estrogens for acne, birth control, and then later in life for premenopause, and menopause, but we are also exposed to estrogen-like compounds in the form of xeno-estrogens and phyto-estrogens (see page 249). All of these synthetic estrogens have strongly contributed to the risks of endometrial cancer, breast cancer, and stroke. We have created diseases as a result of synthetic estrogen overload. Other medications, like natural progesterone cream are required to overcome the effects of the excess estrogens to which we are exposed. Doctors finally realized that excess estrogen can lead to serious medical problems if not balanced by use of another hormone, progesterone. However, instead of adding natural progesterone, pharmaceutical companies created synthetic forms which not only do not effectively counteract the effects of estrogen, but cause its own set of serious problems.

Understanding the serious side effects of these synthetic estrogen and progesterone hormones is crucial to lowering the risk of cancer, heart disease, stroke, etc. You must control exposure to synthetic hormones, thereby reducing the incidence of these serious diseases.

The birth control pill is unavoidably dangerous, hormone replacement therapy is unavoidably dangerous. A majority of women in our society suffer from insufficient progesterone because of their high intake of estrogens and estrogen mimicking substances. The answer to these problems is not additional progesterone, but the stopping of the intake of excess estrogen. If you are taking the birth control pill, stop. If you are taking hormone replacement therapy, stop. If the doctor prescribes the birth control pill for your teen age daughter for acne or to regulate her menstrual cycle, find another doctor. Life is not a disease that needs to be chemically balanced by synthetic products.

ଔଓଔଓ

SCIENTIFIC LITERATURE REVIEW

The scientific literature refutes the belief that synthetic hormone replacement therapy protects against cardiac and osteoporosis diseases.

ରେ ରେ ରେ ରେ
Hormone Replacement Therapy Study
Questions Heart Benefits

ROCHESTER, Minnesota (MAYO CLINIC) - A new study raises questions about the cardiovascular benefits of estrogen-progestin hormone replacement therapy (HRT) in older women who already have heart disease.

A study of more than 2,700 middle-age and older women by Curt Furberg, M.D., of Wake Forest University, Winston-Salem, N.D., and colleagues found that daily use of an estrogen-progestin pill did not reduce the incidence of death or heart attack.

Dr. Furberg and colleagues found that those taking the estrogen-progestin pill actually had a higher risk of heart attacks and death during the first year than did those on the placebo, but had a lower risk during the final 2 years of the study.

The research raises questions about previous observational studies indicating that women on HRT have fewer heart attacks. The latest findings also raise questions about whether the apparent short-term risk of beginning hormone replacement therapy is offset by its potential long-term benefits.

"Based on the binding of no overall cardiovascular benefit and a pattern of early increase in risk of (coronary heart disease) events, we do not recommend starting this treatment for the purpose of secondary prevention of (coronary heart disease)," the authors conclude.

A cautionary note:

"There are two findings here that we should be cautious about," says <u>Brooks S. Edwards, M.D.,</u> a cardiologist at Mayo Clinic, Rochester, Minn. "First, there seems to be an increase in cardiac events in the early period of hormone replacement therapy in women with coronary disease. Maybe the message here is, IF you have an unstable situation, maybe you shouldn't be introducing hormones at that time."

"Second, women in the study had an increase of venous thrombosis (blood clots) forming in the leg that sometimes traveled to the lung and caused damage," Dr. Edwards says. "Patients need to be aware of that risk too."

ଓଲ୍ଡଓଲ୍ଡ

Hormone Therapy No Help For Heart Disease Prevention
WASHINGTON (Reuters) - August 18, 1998.

"I think that certainly women SHOULDN'T start taking it for the purpose of preventing heart disease because there's no proof that it works," Dr. Jacques Rossouw, who is conducting a similar, longer-term study at the National Heart, Lung and Blood Institute (NHLBI), said in a telephone interview.

ଓଲ୍ଡଓଲ୍ଡ

ACC Report: Estrogen May Have Adverse Effects in Postmenopausal Women with CAD

NEW ORLEANS (Reuters Health) - March 11, 1999.

Duke investigators warned their colleagues here in attendance at the 48th annual meeting of the American College of Cardiology that initiation of estrogen replacement therapy may actually increase the incidence of cardiac events in postmenopausal women with established coronary artery disease.

Dr. Karen P. Alexander presented data on more than 1,850 women with a history of myocardial infarction, who were enrolled in a 1996 study of the cardio-protective effects of aspirin. She reported that more than 37% of women who began hormone replacement therapy after study enrollment were hospitalized with unstable angina within one year. In contrast, the hospitalization rate for women who had never used hormone replacement therapy was 17% and the rate for those already on hormone replacement therapy prior to aspirin therapy was 21%, Dr. Alexander told meeting participants.

The study results are similar to those reported last summer by a team at the University of California at San Francisco, Dr. Alexander said. In the earlier study, among women with heart disease who began estrogen replacement therapy after beginning either aspirin or coumadin to prevent reinfarction, nearly one third were hospitalized with unstable angina within a year. By comparison, the hospitalization rate was 21% in those already on estrogen prior to starting either aspirin or coumadin.

"While hormone use has benefits and may still be cardio-protective in women without heart disease, women who have heart disease should probably not start using [hormones]," Dr. Alexander said in a university statement. "We also have no reason to suggest women stop using hormones if they develop heart disease."

CRCRCRCR

HRT and Prevention of Coronary Heart Disease (CHD)
Excerpts from Dr. Lee's Newsletter

It is widely advertised that conventional HRT should be given to all postmenopausal women to prevent coronary heart disease. But is there good evidence for this claim? The reference most widely used to claim a heart benefit from HRT is the Nurses Questionnaire study, which was neither randomized, nor placebo controlled. A critique of this study appears in chapter 13 of Dr. Lee's book, "What Your Doctor May Not Tell You About Menopause" (see References). Recently JAMA published a randomized blinded study of 2,763 postmenopausal women followed for five years. One half of the women received Premarin 0.625 mg and Provera 2.5 mg. daily; and the other half received placebo. After five years of follow-up, there was no evidence of a cardiac benefit from hormone therapy. There was, however, a three-fold increase in the incidence of thromboembolic events [blood clots in the legs and lungs] and a significant increase in gallbladder disease in the treatment group compared to controls.

Similarly, the long-running Framingham study has compared the incidence of coronary heart disease with postmenopausal hormone replacement therapy and found no correlation.

If evidence-based medicine is your guide, the claim that HRT prevents CHD must be discarded.

ೞೞೞೞ

PHYSICIANS' COMMITTEE FOR RESPONSIBLE MEDICINE
Estrogen Replacement Not Advisable For Osteoporosis, Heart Disease
David Wasser, Media Director June 20, 1995

So why are so many doctors prescribing Hormone Replacement Therapy? Most of the push relates to osteoporosis and heart disease. Osteoporosis is very common in Caucasian women, less so among other races. About a quarter of white women over sixty have compression fractures of their vertebrae, and many develop hip fractures due to the gradual loss of bone. But estrogens are not nearly as good at protecting the bones as women may be led to believe, and they rarely arrest bone loss. At best, estrogens simply slow the rate of bone deterioration. Other approaches are much more effective, and they do not cause cancer. For example, a major article in the American Journal of Clinical Nutrition reported that eliminating meat from the diet can cut urinary calcium losses in half. This supports other studies showing that populations that follow plant-based diets have enviably low rates of hip fracture. Cutting salt intake can reduce calcium losses even further. Limiting caffeine consumption will hold onto still more calcium, and if patients don't smoke, they will avoid the 10% loss of bone that plagues chronic smokers.

For heart disease prevention, hormones are no match for lifestyle changes. But Americans want pills, and they don't want to be told to change their diets. According to PCRM, that's nonsense. It is patronizing to assume that every postmenopausal woman is too wedded to her current diet and lifestyle to listen to competent advice. The real problem is, she is not likely to find such advice. Most doctors know little about how diet affects health, even when a mountain of research has already been done, and is gathering dust in medical libraries. They rely instead on knee-jerk prescribing, which is continually encouraged by drug manufacturers' aggressive promotions. When doctors learn how to use all the tools their medical bags could really offer--including prescriptions for diet and lifestyle changes, their patients will be much better off.

For additional information or membership, contact PCRM at: PCRM 5100 Wisconsin Avenue, Suite 404 Washington, DC 20016 Phone: (202) 686-2210 FAX: (202) 686-2216

ଔଓଔଓ

Here are some interesting medical statistics:

Taking [synthetic] estrogen for 10 years increases the probability of developing breast cancer to about 10.7%; taking [synthetic] estrogen for 15 years may increase it to 13%, and has a 15% lifetime probability of having an osteoporotic hip fracture and a 1.5% probability of death from hip fracture. The median age of women for hip fracture is 79 years. This information is from "Menopause: Epidemiologic Aspects" by William R. Harlan, in Women's Health in Menopause, edited by P.G. Crosignani et al, Kluwer Academic Publishers, 1994.

ଔଓଔଓ

Synthetic Hormone Replacement Therapy

REFERENCES

Berger, Gary S., M.D., <u>The Couples' Guide to Infertility</u>, 1995.

Couple to Couple League's website is <u>http://www.ccli.org</u>

Epstein, Steinman, LeVert, <u>The Breast Cancer Prevention Program</u>,"Chapter 3, The Pill: Assessing Your Risks." Macmillan, U.S.A.

http://www.homefirst.com (The Homefirst® WEB page containing extensive links to research on "the Pill", as well as many related topics).

Lee, M.D., John R., <u>What Your Doctor May *Not* Tell You about PREMENOPAUSE</u>, (Balancing Your Hormones and Your Life From Thirty to Fifty) Warner Books, 1999. Women considering synthetic hormone replacement therapy (HRT) for menopause symptoms and health benefits should read this book first. Lee has studied the research and concludes that estrogen is not the magic bullet for protection against heart disease and osteoporosis, nor does it retard aging. Natural progesterone, instead, puts postmenopausal women's hormones in balance. Dr. Lee cites study after study that indicates that natural progesterone, obtained in cream form, delivers what the synthetic HRT only promises.

Lee, M.D., John. <u>What Your Doctor May Not Tell You About Menopause: The Breakthrough Book on Natural Progesterone</u>, 1996.

Martin, Gerstung. <u>The Estrogen Alternative: Natural Hormone Therapy With Botanical Progesterone</u>, Healing Arts Press, 1998.

Mintz, Morton <u>The Pill An Alarming Report</u>,(*Washington Post)* 1969.

Ratner, Herbert, M.D., <u>The Medical Hazards of the Birth Control Pill</u>, "Child and Family" 1970.

Seaman, Barbara, <u>The Doctor's Case Against the Pill</u>, 1995 (original publication 1969), Hunter House.

Theo Colborn, et al, <u>Our Stolen Future</u>, Penguin Group, 1997.

Wright, Jonathan, V., M.D., <u>Natural Hormone Replacement For Women Over 45</u>; Smart Publications, 1997.

Chapter X

Estrogen the Common
Link to Breast Cancer

Estrogen is intimately connected to the development of most breast cancers. Estrogen encourages breast cells to divide more often and more rapidly. Thus, if a mutation (inherited or triggered by a carcinogen) lies imbedded in the DNA, cancer cells are more likely to proliferate when high estrogen levels are present. (The main reason that men, who also have breasts and breast tissue, rarely develop breast cancer is that their exposure to estrogen is minimal.) This also may help to explain why breast cancer rates in women have increased in tandem with the widespread use of birth control pills and estrogen replacement therapy, both of these increase the amount of estrogen circulating in a woman's body. Indeed, we now know that two distinct types of breast cancer exist: the far more common, estrogen-dependent breast cancer influenced primarily by estrogen, and the less common, non-estrogen dependent breast cancer. More than 2/3 of women with breast cancer have estrogen-dependent cancers, and that number is increasing at a particularly alarming rate. According to a study published in 1990 by the Journal of the National Cancer Institute, the incidence of estrogen-dependent breast cancers, particularly among post-menopausal women, increased by 130% from mid-1970's to the mid-1980's in contrast to only a 27% increase in non-estrogen-dependent cancers. A 1997 study in the same journal confirmed these findings.

Contrary to what you may have heard or read, oral contraceptives ("the Pill"), and Hormone Replacement Therapy do not protect against heart disease, they do cause increased blood clots, cancer, strokes, etc. and there are other safer means to prevent osteoporosis. Estrogen replacement therapy is an avoidable cause of breast cancer. Risks are greatest with prolonged use and high doses and also with estrogen-progestin combinations."

The birth control pills: first, second and third generations are avoidably dangerous drugs. With every subsequent generation of birth control pills the dangers did not decline. Birth control pills are contraindicated especially for women with benign breast disease, with a family history of breast cancer, or who began taking oral contraceptives in their teen years.

Doctors and the public have been indoctrinated as to the medicinal value of the birth control pill. Doctors believe that pregnancy is a disease to be avoided and that menopause is a fate worse than death. They now have a reason to dose a woman with estrogen from her reproductive years through menopause. Doctors continue to ignore the growing body of evidence as to the risk of synthetic hormones. Even when the evidence demonstrates a very strong association between synthetic estrogens and breast and endometrial cancers, doctors refuse to change their position. They argue that synthetic estrogens are still valuable because they lower the incidence of heart disease and osteoporosis in women. These arguments have not been scientifically validated.

There is no benefit in taking synthetic estrogens to prevent heart disease. The benefits that synthetic hormones allegedly have in preventing osteoporosis are not only questionable but the same or better results can be obtained by diet, exercise and the application of the safe, natural progesterone creams.

಄ರ಄ಡ

A Survey of the Scientific Literature

Estrogen, Abortion and Cancer

National Right to Life News - August 12, 1997

Estradiol (one of the bodies natural estrogens) increases 20 times higher during the first trimester of pregnancy. If the pregnancy is completed the growth of breast tissue is halted and replaced with milk producing tissues. Thus, if pregnancy is stopped short by abortion, or breast feeding is not used, the excess estrogen level in blood may promote breast tissue to grow abnormally into cancerous cells.

Chapter X - Page 233

Pregnancies which terminate spontaneously or naturally are associated with low estrogen levels and thus do not present the problem of excess estrogen stimulation.

ෆ෪෪෪

Birth Control Pills (Synthetic Estrogen Hormones)
http:/www.web.tusco.net/newone/estrogen.htm

Birth control pills usually contain about .1 mg. of synthetic estrogen and about 2 mg. of synthetic progesterone. The administration of birth control pills prevents the female body from producing the natural hormones resulting in no egg formation or not further development of a fertilized egg (a chemically induced abortion). Natural estrogen and natural progesterone metabolize or oxidize quickly and there to be effective as contraceptives they have to be administered via injection or transdermally. Synthetic analogs, which have slightly different chemical structures, do not metabolize or oxidize quickly and thus could be used in pill form. Unfortunately, the synthetic hormones can accumulate in the human body in very high dosages. The level of natural estrogen in the adult body is about 2 to 20 ppt (parts per trillion). The .1 mg. found in birth control pills amounts to about 300,000 ppt for a woman who weighs 160 pounds.

Doses of xeno-estrogen (such as DDT, PCBs which act like human estrogen) chemicals at 2,000 parts ppt are already enough to produce abnormality in the reproductive system of clinical rats. RU 486, the abortion inducing chemical, is a synthetic analog of natural progesterone. It has similar chemical structure to natural progesterone but functions much differently. Progesterone is the key hormone in the adult female body which establishes and maintains normal pregnancy. RU486, due to the similar structure, will trick the body to accept it instead of progesterone and due to its high dose the body will stop secreting the natural progesterone hormone which is vital in nurturing the embryo which consequently will die in the uterus. RU486 is recommended to be used for 2 days and 600 mg. level which equals to 10,000,000 ppt or about 1,000,000 times a higher concentration than the normal level in the adult female body.

ରୟରୟ

Synthetic Estrogen and the
Natural Toxicology Program

http:/www.web.tusco.net/newone/estrogen.htm

Every two years the Natural Toxicology Program (NTP) of Department of Health and Human Services (HHS) publishes a list of carcinogens, dividing them into two categories. One, substances known to be human carcinogens. Two, substances reasonably anticipated to be human carcinogens. The 1994 NTP Report included the following as carcinogens: conjugated estrogens; DES, progesterone, estrone, mestranol, ethinylestradiol. Some of these naturally occurring hormones are practically safe at minute levels (ppt). However, if these hormones, especially the synthetic ones, are introduced into human bodies as contraceptive and abortion chemicals at such massive doses as the ones in birth control pills or RU486, many dangerous side effects, including cancers to both mothers and her offspring might occur. In 1989 the European Community banned all US beef which is produced with growth hormones, i.e. synthetic estrogens, since they deemed the products potentially cancerous. The residual levels of synthetic hormones in this U.S. beef was measured at about 600 - 1,000 ppt. However, the same Europeans are still taking daily birth control pills which contain much higher levels

Chapter X - Page 236

of synthetic estrogen than US beef. The level in birth control pills is estimated to be 100 - 1,000 times higher than in U.S. beef grown with synthetic hormones.

The increased infertility in Western women is possibly due, in part, to their artificially high levels of synthetic estrogen. The cancer rate in Japan, which is much lower than other industrial countries, may not be due to the soy products they eat but due to the fact that the birth control pill, until recently, has been banned in Japan.

It is now evident that estrogen can induce cancerous growths in reproductive systems at very minute levels. Every year there are 150,000 children born with severe birth defects possibly due to the exogenous hormones which their mothers have ingested knowingly and unknowingly. The adverse effects of synthetic estrogen can be permanent and irreversible for both mother and her offspring, even if a woman only took birth control pills for six months or less. When being exposed to a continuously high level of hormones, the body and its reproductive system might be altered and adapt to those extremely high levels of artificial hormones. The body might continue to respond only to the high levels of hormones, but not to the much lower levels which previously existed. That may mean that the body may need artificially induced high levels of estrogen or estrogen like compounds in order for the reproductive system to function normally.

ଔଔଔଔ

Estrogen and Breast Cancer
New England Journal of Medicine 2/27/97...
CNN Internet
New Study Links Estrogen Treatment and
Breast Cancer

"The new report in the *NEJM* gives women plenty to think about. When researchers tracked 1300 women for 25 years, they found that those who had the most dense bones were 3.5 times more likely to develop breast cancer than those with the least dense bones. The researchers say a woman's bone mass may be a way of measuring her estrogen exposure over time. Knowing her estrogen exposure may help to predict her risk of breast cancer... The researchers also say it may be a woman's lifetime exposure to estrogen that would increase her chances of developing breast cancer – not necessarily estrogen taken during and after menopause."

ଔଔଔଔ

The Harvard Nurses Health Study - July 1997

The recent update from the *Harvard Nurses Health Study* has linked the long-term effects of HRT with breast cancer. The Harvard study which followed 121,700 nurses found that HRT for five or more years after menopause increased a woman's breast cancer risk by 30% if she takes estrogen alone and 40% if she's on estrogen and progestin

೮ೞೞೞ

"Menopause" - 1998 Fall; 5(3): 145-51, Brinton, LA

Breast cancer risk among women under 55 years of age by joint effects of usage of oral contraceptives and hormone replacement therapy.

A case control study of breast cancer among women under the age of 55 years in was held in Atlanta, Georgia. Results: Use of oral contraceptives was associated with a relative risk of 1.1 whereas the relative risk for hormone replacement therapy was .9. When the combined effects of longer use of both agents were considered, subjects who reported use of oral contraceptives for 10 or more years and hormone replacement for 3 or more years had a relative risk of 3.2 compared with non-users of either preparation. (A relative risk of 3.2 means it is 320 times more likely than the non-user population.)

Conclusion: This study raises the necessity of further evaluation of breast cancer risk from the increase in the common exposure to both oral contraceptives and hormone replacement therapy.

 CRCRCRCR

HRT Link to Breast Cancer Risk

Journal of the National Cancer Institute, 1998; 90:814-823, Dr. Graham Colditz of Harvard Medical School in Boston, Massachusetts.

Hormone replacement therapy appears to increase the risk of breast cancer in post-menopausal women, according to a review of available data published in the "Journal of the American Cancer Institute". An analysis of 51 studies involving more than 150,000 women with and without breast cancer found that each year of hormone use increased the risk of breast cancer by 2.3%.

CRCRCRCR

High Level of Estrogen Increases Breast Cancer Risk for Postmenopausal Women

<u>"Journal National Cancer Institute"</u>
<u>1998;90:1292-1299</u>, Dr. Susan E.
Hankinson, of Harvard Medical School,
Boston, Mass.

"A high plasma level of estrogen is associated with an increased risk of breast cancer among postmenopausal women, according to the results of a case controlled study conducted as part of the nurses health study."

ଓଷଓଷ

Hormone Replacement Therapy Linked to Increase in Breast Tissue Density

"Annals Internal Medicine" 1999;130:262-269. Dr. Elizabeth Barrett-Connor, of the University of California San Diego

"Hormone replacement therapy, particularly estrogen-progestin regiments, significantly increases mammographic density in the first year of use, potentially increasing the risk of breast cancer."

ଓଷଓଷ

Hormone Replacement Therapy and Risk for Breast Cancer

Endocrinology and Metabolism Clinics Vol. 26, No. 2, June 1997, Louis A. Brinton, Ph.D., Environmental Epidemiology Branch, National Cancer Institute.

"An influence of estrogens on breast cancer was acknowledged as early as 1886 when a palliative effect of oopherectomy on advanced breast cancer was described... Menopausal estrogens have become one of the most widely used drugs. An estimated 31.7 million prescriptions for oral medications were dispensed in 1992."

ଓଃଔଓଔ

Menopausal Estrogen and Estrogen-Progestin Replacement Therapy and Breast Cancer Risk

JAMA Vol. 283 No. 4, January 2000, Schairer, Catherine, et al.

"Using estrogen combined with progesterone for hormone replacement therapy (HRT) for more than a few years increases a woman's risk of breast cancer far beyond that she would experience without the therapy [HRT]..."

The study reported in the January 26, 2000 *Journal of the American Medical Association* involved over 46,000 women. Compared with women who received no hormone therapy, women who took estrogen and progesterone in combination for an average of 3.5 years had a 40% greater chance of developing breast cancer. The risks were also calculated based on each subsequent year of use. Women on estrogen alone had an increased risk of 1% a year for each year of use, compared with the women on the estrogen-progesterone combination, for whom the increase was 8% a year. [Editor's note: the estrogen in all of these studies is synthetic, not natural estrogen and the progesterone, is not natural progesterone it is a synthetic progestin].

ೞೞೞೞ
Estrogen & Breast Cancer - A Warning to Women,
Rinzler, CarolAnn, Hunter House, 1996
(page 170-171).

...throughout the 1980's as the incidence of breast cancer in the United States continued to rise, American women and their doctors searched for a reasonable explanation for the epidemic... The explanation is this: Exposure to estrogen-both the estrogen produced in a woman's body and the [synthetic] estrogen she takes in a variety of drugs - increases the risk of breast cancer... In the end we must accept the evidence before our eyes without fear or prejudice. It is our only hope for defeating this disease.

ଔଙ୍ଔଙ୍

REFERENCES

Berger, Gary S. Dr. ,The Couples' Guide to Infertility, 1995.

Couple to Couple League's website is http://www.ccli.org

Epstein, Steinman, LeVert, The Breast Cancer Prevention Program, - "Chapter 3, The Pill: Assessing Your Risks" Macmillan, U.S.A.

Lee, John M.D., What Your Doctor May Not Tell You About Menopause: The Breakthrough Book on Natural Progesterone, 1996.

Lee, M.D., John R., What Your Doctor May *Not* Tell You about PREMENOPAUSE, (Balancing Your Hormones and Your Life From Thirty to Fifty) Warner Books, 1999.
Women considering synthetic hormone replacement therapy (HRT) for menopause symptoms and health benefits should read this book first. Lee has studied the research and concludes that estrogen is not the magic bullet for protection against heart disease and osteoporosis, nor does it retard aging. Natural progesterone, instead, puts postmenopausal women's hormones in balance. Dr. Lee cites study after study that indicates that natural progesterone, obtained in cream form, delivers what the synthetic HRT only promises.

Martin, Gerstung, The Estrogen Alternative: Natural Hormone Therapy With Botanical Progesterone, Healing Arts Press, 1998.

Mintz, Morton "The Pill An Alarming Report," <u>Washington Post</u> 1969.

Ratner, Herbert M.D., "The Medical Hazards of the Birth Control Pill," <u>Child and Family</u> 1970.

Rinzler, CarolAnn, <u>Estrogen & Breast Cancer - A Warning to Women</u>, Hunter House, 1996.
Why breast cancer has reached epidemic proportions. How HRT and th Pill have contributed to its rise. What women and their doctors can do to reduce the risks.

Schairer, Catherine, et al, JAMA Vol. 283 No. 4, 2000 "Menopausal Estrogen and Estrogen-Progestin Replacement Therapy and Breast Cancer Risk"

Seaman, Barbara <u>The Doctor's Case Against the Pill</u>, 1995 (original publication 1969), Hunter House.

Wright, M.D., Jonathan, V. <u>Natural Hormone Replacement For Women Over 45</u>; Smart Publications, 1997.

www.homefirst.com (The Homefirst® WEB page containing extensive links to research on the "Pill", as well as many related topics).

Chapter XI

Natural Progesterone Cream
for women

Scientific studies have shown that many of the following symptoms and conditions may be caused by hormonal imbalance because of excess estrogen ingestion and alleviated by the simple use of a totally safe transdermal natural progesterone cream applied twice daily for three to six months.

- breast tenderness
- cervical dysplasia
- decreased sex drive
- depression
- endometriosis
- fat gain - especially around the abdomen, hips & thighs
- fatigue

- fibrocystic breasts
- fibroids
- headaches
- hot flashes
- infertility
- insomnia
- irregular menstrual periods
- migraine headaches
- miscarriages

- mood swings
- night sweats
- osteoporosis
- PMS
- skin conditions (i.e. acne, seborrhea, Rosaceae, psoriasis, keratosis)
- water retention
- vaginal dryness

The timing during your menstrual cycle and the amount of natural progesterone cream that you need to use to reduce EOS (estrogen overload syndrome) will depend and vary with the different symptoms that you are experiencing. Detailed information is available at www.homefirst.com or by calling any of the Homefirst® offices.

WHY SO MUCH ESTROGEN?

The body regulates the production of estrogen and progesterone, however, we are exposed to so many extraneous sources of estrogen that the female endocrine system cannot maintain the hormones in balance. Many young, middle aged and elderly women suffer from symptoms that are brought about by estrogen overload thus requiring supplemental progesterone to achieve hormone balance.

Sources of Estrogen

1) Natural estrogen - produced by your body.
2) Synthetic estrogen (i.e. birth control pills, estrogen replacement therapies). The pharmaceutical industry has developed a wide variety of synthetic estrogens more potentially carcinogenic, which stay in the body longer than the natural estrogens. Ethanol estradiol is used in the birth control pills and is one example of a synthetic estrogen. Prolonged exposure to synthetic estrogen significantly increases the risk for developing breast cancer and EOS.

3) Xeno-estrogens, also known as pseudo-estrogens, are synthetic chemicals in products such as pesticides, plastic, solvents, adhesives, car exhaust, industrial waste (i.e. PCBs and dioxins) and in meat from livestock fed estrogenic drugs to fatten them up. These xeno-estrogens exert hormonal influences on all living creatures by disrupting reproductive abilities and hormonal balance. Several dietary contaminants, industrial chemicals and insecticides mimic estrogen. Although chemically quite different from estrogen, they affect menstrual and reproductive cycles as well as triggering both normal and abnormal cell division.

4) Phyto-estrogens (plant derived). Certain plants contain substances that have estrogenic effects in the body. Some phyto-estrogens (i.e. soybeans, tofu), stimulate the production of estrogen; however, other phyto-estrogens such as zeranol, which is found in some fungi, and used to fatten cattle, can disrupt the body's balance of estrogen, placing one into EOS (estrogen overload syndrome) and producing all its potential problems.

WHY DO MANY WOMEN NEED SUPPLEMENTAL PROGESTERONE?

All estrogen, without the balance of progesterone, will increase cell proliferation, can be a precursor or cause of cancer (breast, uterus, cervix, ovaries, etc.) and can cause EOS.

We are living in a sea of estrogen. From the birth control pill to hormone replacement therapy HRT to synthetic chemicals to phyto-estrogens, we ingest estrogen from youth to grave. Environmental and food sources which contain high levels of estrogen like compounds may cause symptoms of EOS (estrogen overload syndrome), even if you never used the birth control pill or HRT. The use of a natural progesterone will curtail the cellular proliferation effects of estrogen.

WHY NATURAL PROGESTERONE??... *OR* WHY SYNTHETIC PROGESTERONE HAS NOT SOLVED THE PROBLEM OF EOS ?

About 50 years ago scientists discovered that the Mexican wild yam contains substances which are chemically similar to human progesterone. Through fermentation and other steps in the laboratory scientists converted this substance into a molecular structure **identical** to the progesterone produced by the human body.

Doctors have begun to recognize the potential problems of hormone imbalance. To solve this problem they have added synthetic progesterone to the birth control pill as well as to the hormone replacement therapy regimens. However, these synthetic progesterone hormones (i.e. Provera, Depo-Provera, progestins) are all poorly absorbed, do not have the effect of countering the effects of estrogen hormones and cause many serious side effects. These synthetic chemicals have been linked to many serious side-effects. A partial listing from the PDR [Physicians Desk Reference] includes high blood pressure, blood clots in the lung and brain, headaches, changes in libido, fatigue, hirsutism, hemorrhagic eruptions and coagulation problems. **Natural progesterones work without any of the serious side effects of the synthetic progesterones.** Products such as natural progesterone cannot be patented. The pharmaceutical companies, in order to patent their designer progestin products, must alter the natural progesterone.

What To Do

If you are taking the birth control pill **stop**. If you are taking synthetic hormone replacement therapy drugs (i.e. Premarin, Provera) see a physician who understands the concept of EOS and will help you with a natural program that will restore your hormonal balance. Natural progesterone cream can actually help achieve hormone balance. Natural progesterone cream is absorbed through the skin and can act to reverse many of the EOS symptoms. Natural progesterone cream is not altered by the liver to create other potentially harmful compounds.

Are All Natural Progesterone Creams The Same

Not all natural progesterone creams have the same amount of natural progesterone. The dosage may be too low or too high. They range from as little as 100 mg. per ounce to 1,000 mg. per ounce. The physiologic dose is approximately 30-40 mg. per day.

Some products are actually wild yam extracts which may be progestin, a compound similar to, but not the equivalent of, natural progesterone. Be sure that the natural progesterone cream that you use falls into the proper category. Also, some products will contain other ingredients which may hinder or alter absorption.

QUESTIONS & ANSWERS

Q. Do I need to see a physician to be on a program of natural progesterone cream?

A. No, natural progesterone cream is not a prescription item. However, it is advisable to have a consultation with a physician who is well versed in the issue of natural vs. synthetic hormone treatment. That physician will be able to advise you on the proper application and dosage.

Q. Can my estrogen and progesterone levels be measured?

A. Yes, the most accurate method for testing hormones, such as estrogen and progesterone, is through the saliva (not with a blood test).

Q. Is it necessary to test my hormone levels?

A. In most cases hormone balance can be achieved without measuring the levels. The disappearance of symptoms with the use of natural progesterone cream will tell you that your hormones are in balance even without knowing the specific levels.

Q. Is there a time limit on how long I can use natural progesterone cream?

A. No. However, if you become asymptomatic you may want to consult with your physician on the proper dosage.

Q. How long until I see results?

A. Results will vary, however, usually you will see some results within two to three weeks.

Q. My doctor says that I have fibroids and should have a hysterectomy. Will natural progesterone cream help?

A. Many times fibroids are caused by EOS (estrogen overload syndrome) and will shrink with the use of natural progesterone cream.

Q. My doctor says that I have polycystic ovarian (POS) syndrome. Will natural progesterone cream help?

A. Many times POS prevents ovulation and thereby prevents the natural production of progesterone. Therefore, using natural progesterone cream helps to restore the proper hormonal balance.

Q. My physician says that I have endometriosis. Will natural progesterone cream help?

A. Endometriosis has many possible causes. If the cause is hormone imbalance, the natural progesterone cream will help.

Q. I have been diagnosed with PMS. Will natural progesterone cream help?

A. If the PMS is caused by hormone imbalance, natural progesterone cream will help.

Q. Before my period my breasts are lumpy and painful. What can I do?

A. This condition is known as fibrocystic breast disease. It is sometimes caused by hormone imbalance and can be helped with natural progesterone cream.

Q. I am experiencing hot flashes and my doctor told me I need estrogen to control these symptoms.

A. Many times progesterone will alleviate hot flashes without any side effects. Before trying a trial of estrogen, I would recommend natural progesterone cream.

Q. Can natural progesterone cream help with PMS, EOS (estrogen overload syndrome) endometriosis or fibrocystic breast disease?

A. Yes, because progesterone is the precursor hormone helping to normalize all other endocrine and hormonal activity in the body. It assists in lowering the level of estrogen in the body, thus helping to alleviate these diseases and achieve hormone balance. Research has shown that women with PMS, endometriosis, or fibrocystic breast disease tend to have lower progesterone levels and 90% of these women can be successfully treated with natural progesterone.

Q. Does natural progesterone cream help vaginal dryness?

A. Yes, natural hormones in a cream base can be used intra-vaginally and can be used in treating vaginal dryness and vulvar atrophy associated with aging.

Q. I am already taking *synthetic hormone replacement therapy (Premarin, Provera) from my doctor, can I switch to natural progesterone cream?*

A. Absolutely yes. It is advisable, however, to consult with a physician familiar with natural progesterone treatment. Natural hormones are simply a safe alternative to hormone replacement therapy. Synthetic hormones have many side effects and can be dangerous to your health.

Q. Where should the natural progesterone cream be applied?

A. Morning and night to areas of soft skin such as the face, hands, chest, breast, inner arms, soles of feet. Periodically apply to different areas of the skin. The cream is readily absorbed and leaves no trace after a few minutes.

Q. Are there any other benefits of natural progesterone cream use?

A. Additional benefits which have been reported include: improved brain function, improved sleep pattern, diminished muscular aches and pains, improvement of skin problems, including acne, seborrhea, Rosacea, psoriasis and keratosis.

Q. Will I experience any problems when I start using natural progesterone cream?

A. Most women will experience no side effects from natural progesterone. However, in premenopausal women who have been progesterone deficient for years, it is common that the initial application of progesterone will cause water retention, headaches, and swollen breasts, symptoms of estrogen dominance. This happens because the estrogen receptors shut down by progesterone deficiency are waking up. It is important to remember that these symptoms will disappear in two week to 2-3 months.

Q. Can I use too much natural progesterone cream?

A. Yes, it contains an active hormone. Even though there are no known side effects from the use of natural progesterone cream, it is important to use the proper range of dosage. If you start to experience symptoms such as - tiredness and lethargy, you are most probably using too much.

REFERENCES

Lee, M.D., John. <u>What Your Doctor May Not Tell You About Menopause: The Breakthrough Book on Natural Progesterone</u>, 1996.

Lee, M.D., John R., <u>What Your Doctor May *Not* Tell You about PREMENOPAUSE</u>, (Balancing Your Hormones and Your Life From Thirty to Fifty) Warner Books, 1999.

   Women considering synthetic hormone replacement therapy (HRT) for menopause symptoms and health benefits should read this book first. Lee has studied the research and concludes that estrogen is not the magic bullet for protection against heart disease and osteoporosis, nor does it retard aging. Natural progesterone, instead, puts postmenopausal women's hormones in balance. Dr. Lee cites study after study that indicates that natural progesterone, obtained in cream form, delivers what the synthetic HRT only promises.

Martin, Gerstung, <u>The Estrogen Alternative: Natural Hormone Therapy With Botanical Progesterone</u>, Healing Arts Press, 1998.

Wright, M.D., Jonathan, V. <u>Natural Hormone Replacement For Women Over 45</u>; Smart Publications, 1997.

<u>www.homefirst.com</u> Detailed information is presented regarding dosage and usage of natural progesterone cream. Also contains multiple links to other valuable sites with scientific information about natural progesterone cream.

Natural Progesterone Cream
for men

Benign Prostatic Hypertrophy
(Non-Cancerous Enlargement of the Prostate)

The following are some of the symptoms that have been associated with BPH:

- straining to start a urinary stream
- a weak urinary stream
- dribbling of urine
- dysuria - painful urination
- incomplete emptying of bladder leading to cystitis
- discomfort during intercourse
- painful ejaculation
- impotence
- lowered sex drive
- the need to urinate frequently
- lower back pain

Somewhere between the ages of 30 and 40 a man's prostate begins to enlarge. The growth of the prostate is known as Benign Prostatic Hypertrophy (BPH). BPH will affect nearly all men as they age. What is generally not known is the fact that there are safe, natural and effective ways of dealing with BPH. By age 50 more than 50% of men will have prostate surgery, radiation treatment, or will be on prescription drugs like Proscar (finasteride). Finasteride has been shown to cause impotence in more than 60% of patients [*Physician's Desk Reference - PDR®*, Medical Economics, 2000], decreased libido, decreased amount of semen per ejaculation, breast tenderness, breast enlargement, lip swelling and skin rashes.

Scientific studies have shown that many of the symptoms of BPH may be alleviated by a combination of a natural progesterone cream applied twice a day, along with herbal vitamin and mineral pills which include some or all of the following: Saw Palmetto Berry (Serenoa Repens), Pygeum Africanum, American Ginseng (Panax Quinquefolius), Bearberry Extract (Arctostaphylos Uva-Ursi), Pumpkin Seed Oil, Vitamin C, Zinc, Lycopene, Vitamin B6, Magnesium, Stinging Nettle Leaves, Cernilton Flower Pollen, Flaxseed Oil, Evening Primrose Oil, Vitamin E, Copper, Amino Acids, Multi-vitamins and Minerals.

ଽଔଽଔ

Men's Hormones

Progesterone and estradiol (an estrogen) are two hormones naturally produced by the male body, but in smaller amounts than in women and are vital to good health. Progesterone is the primary precursor of adrenal

cortical hormones and testosterone. It also has the effect
of balancing out the effects of estradiol. Uninhibited
estradiol (estradiol without progesterone) has been
implicated in prostate growth leading to BPH. As men age,
their progesterone levels fall, causing their uninhibited
estradiol levels to rise. It has been theorized that one of
the causes of BPH may be inadequate amounts of
progesterone synthesis needed to counteract the effect of
estradiol.

Men also have elevated estrogen levels because of
unavoidable environmental and food sources which contain
high levels of estrogen like compounds. Xeno-estrogens,
also known as pseudo-estrogens, are synthetic chemicals in
products such as pesticides, plastics, solvents, adhesives,
car exhaust, industrial waste (i.e. PCBs and dioxins), meat
from livestock fed estrogenic drugs to fatten them up.
These xeno-estrogens exert estrogen like influences on all
living creatures, male and female, by disrupting the
reproductive abilities and hormonal balance. Several
dietary contaminants, industrial chemicals and insecticides
also act like estrogens.

Since uninhibited estrogen is one of the causes of
enlargement of the prostate and symptoms of BPH, the role
of progesterone is to balance this uninhibited estrogen. **In
fact, natural progesterone may be the only remedy
needed to reverse benign prostatic enlargement.** Men

may also need progesterone to reverse the feminizing effects of too much estrogen.

∽∾∽∾

<u>**Why Natural Progesterone**</u> ??

About 50 years ago scientists discovered that the Mexican wild yam contains substances which are chemically similar to human progesterone. Through fermentation and other steps in the laboratory scientists converted this substance into a molecular structure **identical** to the progesterone produced by the human body.

Products such as natural progesterone cannot be patented. The pharmaceutical companies, in order to patent their designer progestin products (now coming out for men), must alter natural progesterone.   These altered chemicals have been linked to many serious side-effects (a partial listing from the PDR [Physicians Desk Reference] includes high blood pressure, blood clots in the lung and brain, headaches, changes in libido, fatigue, hemorrhagic eruptions, coagulation problems). **Natural progesterones work without any of the serious side effects of the altered synthetic progesterones and do not have any feminizing effect on men.**

∽∾∽∾

Should You Try Alternatives to Surgery & Prescription Medication

Before beginning any hormone treatment, herbal treatment, vitamin treatment, etc. it is advisable to have a thorough medical evaluation to make sure that the genito-urinary problems are due to BPH and not due to infection, bladder stones, or cancer.

கே௧கே௧

<u>Natural Progesterone Cream Dosage and Use</u>

If the doctor determines your symptoms are caused by mild or moderate BPH, it is appropriate to consider natural options before proceeding to pharmaceutical agents or surgery. My recommendation is to begin with a natural progesterone cream, **as this may be the total solution to BPH.** If you still have symptoms, I would begin adding the herbal remedies listed on page 1.

If you decide to use natural progesterone cream, it is important to use one that has the proper amount of natural progesterone. The amount of natural progesterone cream that you need to counteract the estrogenic effect and to cause the prostate to shrink, will depend and vary with the different symptoms that you are experiencing. The recommended physiologic dose for men is 8-12 mg. of

progesterone daily. Detailed information is available at
www.homefirst.com.

The only side effect of natural progesterone cream for
men, mentioned in the literature, is the potential for
decreased sperm motility for men under the age of 35.
This does not mean a decreased number of sperm; it
means that your sperm do not move as quickly. Decreased
motility can either be a positive or a negative depending on
your desire for maximum fertility. There is no evidence
that natural progesterone has any other side effects. Since
BPH and its associated symptoms rarely start before age
40, this side effect will rarely be a significant factor.

CRCRCRCR

Saw Palmetto

Berries from the Saw Palmetto tree have been used to
treat symptoms caused by the enlargement of the prostate
gland, as far back as the Seminole Indians in Florida in the
1700s, according to the report in the November 10, 1998
issue of the Journal of the American Medical Association
(*JAMA*). In the *JAMA* study doctors reviewed 18 studies of
Saw Palmetto use involving 2,939 patients with BPH. Men
taking Saw Palmetto extract were nearly twice as likely to
report improvements in symptoms than men taking
placebos. When compared with Finasteride (Proscar®), a
prescription drug to reduce the size of the prostate, Saw

Palmetto provided similar relief without causing any of the side effects such as impotence. *(Urology* - 1998, Jun; 51(6): 1003-7) "Also, evidence suggests that Saw Palmetto improves urology symptoms and flow measures..." (*JAMA* 1998, Nov. 10; 280(18): 1604-9)

A similar study in the *Journal of Clinical Trials* concluded that Saw Palmetto is a well tolerated agent that may significantly improve lower urinary tract symptoms in men with BPH (*Urology* - 1998 Jun; 51(6): 1003-7).

෩෬෩෬

Lycopene: a Good Reason to Eat Tomatoes

Tomatoes contain numerous nutrients, among them: lycopene. A five year study of 48,000 men found that those eating 10 servings a week of cooked tomato products had the lowest risk of prostate cancer. Their risk was 1/3 that of men eating less than two servings per week. Other studies suggest that lycopene may play a role in reducing the risk of other cancers including colon and rectal cancers. (*Health Oasis Mayo Clinic* - 9/20/98) [http://www.mayohealth.org/mayo/9809/htm/tomato.htm]

෩෬෩෬

Zinc

The ability to absorb zinc declines with age increasing the likelihood of developing BPH. A healthy prostate gland contains more zinc than any other organ in the body. Some experts believe that when zinc is needed in other parts of the body it is taken from the prostate, which is then left with a deficit of this trace mineral.

ೞೞೞೞ

Phyto Medicinals That Show Promise in The Treatment of BPH

Pygeum Africanum and Pumpkin Seed Oil, are among the other phyto-medicinals that have shown promise in the treatment of BPH, without the serious side effects associated with Proscar, surgery, radiation or chemical drugs.

ೞೞೞೞ

Questions and Answers

Q. Do I need to see a physician to be on a program of natural progesterone cream?

A. No, natural progesterone cream is not a prescription item. However, it is advisable to have a consultation with a physician who is well versed in the issue of natural vs.

synthetic hormone treatment. That physician will be able to advise you on the proper application and dosage.

Q. Where should the natural progesterone cream be applied?

A. Morning and night to areas of soft skin such as the face, hands, chest, scrotum, inner arms, soles of feet.
Periodically apply to different areas of the skin. The cream is readily absorbed and leaves no trace after a few minutes.

Q. Is natural progesterone cream for men a feminizing hormone?

A. No, that is the role of estrogen. Remember that in utero all babies (boys and girls) are exposed to high levels of progesterone.

Q. Do men produce progesterone?

A. Yes. The average man produces 8-12 mg. of progesterone per day.

Q. Can natural progesterone cream for men prevent or help BPH?

A. If the BPH is due to exposure to estrogen and estrogen like compounds, the balancing effect of Natural progesterone cream for Men will shrink the prostate and reduce the symptoms.

Q. I get up five to six times a night to urinate. Will natural progesterone cream for men help?

A. If your frequent urination is related to BPH and if the BPH is from EOS natural progesterone cream for men may stop the frequent urination.

REFERENCES FOR PROSTATE HEALTH

Buck, A.C. "Phytotherapy for the Prostate." British Journal of Urology, 78:325-336, 1996.

Lowe, F.C. and J.C. Ku. "Phytotherapy in Treatment of Benign Prostatic Hyperplasia: A Critical Review," Urology 48(1):12-20, 1996.

"Lycopene - a good reason to eat tomatoes." Health Oasis Mayo Clinic, September 1998.

"Saw palmetto extracts for treatment of benign prostatic hyperplasia: a systematic review." JAMA 1998, Nov. 11; 280(18): 1604-9.

"Saw palmetto (Serenoa repens) in men with lower urinary tract symptoms: effects on urodynamic parameters and voiding symptoms." Urology - 1998, Jun; 51(6): 1003-7

www.homefirst.com - Detailed information is presented regarding dosage and usage of natural progesterone cream for men. Also contains multiple links to other valuable sites with scientific information about natural progesterone cream for men.

Chapter XII

Low Carbohydrate Lifestyle

"dieting may be the major cause of obesity"
-Jean-Paul Deslypere,
University of Ghent
Professor of Human Nutrition

I've been on my own diata change. What is diata? It's the Greek word from which the English word diet comes. The root word means lifestyle. For the last thirty years I have tried almost every diet that existed. Every diet concludes its program with the statement **"now that you have reached your goal weight, make a lifestyle change in order to maintain this for the rest of your life"**. I never knew how to accomplish the lifestyle change.

If we could figure it out how to institute the "lifestyle change" we wouldn't have the problem in the first place, and 35% of Americans would not be at least 20% overweight. Ten years ago I thought the answer was to be a vegetarian so I've stopped eating meat and gained about 35 pounds over those ten years. I thought I knew a fair amount about nutrition from being a vegetarian. The one statistic that we all know is that 95% of people who lose more than 30 pounds will gain more than 30 pounds back within the first year after they're off their "diet". The captivation to be thin and slim is so great that we are willing to believe we will be in the less than 5% of the population who will maintain this very thin look. The proliferation of infomercials, one after the other, each promoting a different diet, shows how truly desperate the public is for "the answer". People who have success in most areas - education, business, etc. and who seem to be able to control everything in their life, are the ones who are easiest prey to all the diet gurus who say you just don't have enough self control. That's what they tell them: its your fault. It's a very typical medical philosophy - always blame the victim. After I failed at all the diets, I gave up. I decided that nothing short of "divine intervention" would inspire me to try again.

I have to thank Dr. Paul Schattauer and Dr. Mark Zumhagen, two of my associates, for leaving little hints for something that might help me in this vicious cycle. Six months ago they began their mission. They called me up and said "We want you to buy a book called The Zone by Dr. Barry Sears, and just read the first chapter. You'll like it - it's about sports." Zone (not the title) is a word that's used in sports when everything is going your way - Sosa and McGwire were in the zone during the 1998 and 1999 seasons. Michael Jordan was almost always in the zone.

No matter what you do, you're in the zone so you can't miss.

Dr. Zumhagen then suggested the book called <u>Sugar Busters</u>. Something clicked - could these authors possibly be right? I had to know more. I read Dr. Atkins' book <u>The Diet Revolution</u>. Then I looked at another book just recently published <u>The G Index</u>. G stands for Glycemic Index.

All of the books have a common theme: we've been sold a bill of goods over the last 20 years. What's happened is that we've gone on a low fat diet. The average person in this country is eating 12-15% less fat than they were 20 years ago and the average person is 20% heavier than they were 20 years ago. All of the authors discuss the value of low carbohydrate diets, exactly the opposite of what the

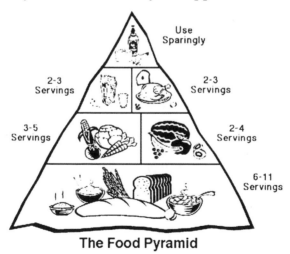

The Food Pyramid

High Carbohydrate Lifestyle Food Pyramid

Chapter XII - Page 273

nutritionists have promoted the last 20 years. Carbohydrates in themselves are not harmful. It is the quantities in which we consume them are way out of proportion to what our body requires. The medical authorities, based on the unscientific USDA food pyramid, have told us to eat a major of our calories from complex carbohydrates, the "good carbohydrates," such as pasta, whole wheat bread, and grains. A more scientific approach would base the food pyramid from a low carbohydrate point of view. My reading put things into perspective and it finally made sense: a vegetarian winds up having way more carbohydrates than anything else in their diet. Take a look at the vegetarian animals, they aren't little animals. They are the elephant, cow, and hippopotamus. Who are the meat eaters? They're the lions, tigers, cats, and dogs. Humans don't have to be meat eaters, but the human physique enables us to. We aren't well put together meat eaters, because our teeth aren't good enough to rip flesh off easily, but we're surely better off than the pure vegetarian ones, the cows and the horses whose teeth are completely flat.

I spent a couple of hours going to grocery stores just looking at the contents of different food. Then I started looking at different menus in restaurants. I would go there just to have a cup of coffee and read the menus. I couldn't get over it. The whole country is in a high carb mode. Just high carb - low fat - that's right - with little symbols like hearts, to indicate good for your heart, after it - low fat + high carb = good heart. Then I looked in the supermarkets and I went even to health minded supermarkets. Is anyone in is tune with this concept of low carbs? The answer is No.

Do low carbs mean high fat? Again, the answer is no! Here is why, if I had 5 pounds of butter, how much of it could anyone eat? If I put oil on the table, I don't care what oils; corn oil, olive oil, or peanut oil, etc., surely you couldn't drink any of it by itself. Fat cannot be consumed unless its mixed with carbohydrates (potatoes, rolls, crackers, etc.). If you lower the fat content of a food, - you must increase something else. That something else is almost always sugar. So all of a sudden it dawned on me – that high carbohydrate/low fat food is the root of the problem. The 20% excess weight of our population didn't come from fruits and vegetables raised in home gardens. The weight came from food bought at food stores, fast food chains, and restaurants.

Essentially, what all of the low carbohydrate authors are saying is that the rise in insulin is what causes the need to consume more and more food. If you know what foods cause a rise in insulin, you're going to be able to control your appetite. The insulin rise from the high carbohydrate meal causes an immediate feeling of being satiated, but then within an hour, as the blood sugar level falls, all of a sudden fatigue sets in and the hunger starts all over again.

Approximately 80% of the population is affected by insulin in this way. Approximately 20% of the population can eat whatever they want and it won't make a difference.

The realization dawned that this was me. Finally, someone was describing what I was experiencing and it made sense. I'd go out for a wonderful dinner and be hungry an hour later. I was eating because of physical hunger, not to fill other needs.

 CRCRCRCR

What Is The Glycemic Index?

The Glycemic Index is the amount of time it takes the insulin to get into the blood stream from the time you ingest the food until there is a rise in blood glucose levels. White bread, with a glycemic index of 100, is the standard. The higher the glycemic index the faster the insulin level is going to rise. A quick rise will cause a quick drop and make you hungrier and fatigued faster. There are two factors which place food lower on the glycemic index. One is fiber and the second one is fat. If a carbohydrate has fiber or fat with it, the glycemic index of that food will be lower. Nuts, which typically have substantial amount of fat and fiber in them, will have a lower glycemic index than white bread which has minimal fiber and fat. Nuts and fruits, in their original state, will have much lower glycemic indices than things like juices which are the fruits with the fiber removed. With the knowledge of the effect of fiber on the glycemic index, for every gram of fiber that you have in your diet, you can eat one more gram of carbohydrate. They essentially cancel each other out. The current trend to feed children fruit juice, a high glycemic index food, contributes to childhood obesity, potentially setting the pattern for a lifetime. It may be one of the reasons why nature made human milk with a higher fat content than cow's milk.

Now popular belief is that grains, especially whole grains are an incredibly good food. There were always candy stores, but now we have boutiques dedicated to single, high carbohydrate foods, i.e. breadshops, potato bars, pasta restaurants, etc. We're talking about life style and diata as opposed to - survival. If the survival is the issue - of course you use grains - because they can be kept for substantial periods of time. We're not talking about foods that are necessarily good or bad for you, but ones that will cause obesity and which aren't necessary in the quantities that we consume them in our society.

Doctors will tell you that a measure of your health is your cholesterol, HDL and triglyceride levels. Let's assume that these indices are predictive of health. You would think that a low fat diet it would work at lowering these three indices. In theory, people who were on a low fat diet would have no need for all these cholesterol lowering and lipid lowering drugs. Just the opposite has proven true. In order to lower these levels you have to have adequate amounts of fats in your diet. Scientific studies have now shown that someone who is on a low carbohydrate diet will have lower HDL, triglyceride and cholesterol levels.

High carbohydrate, low fat diets for weight loss, are the current medical recommendations. In the last decade Americans have reduced their fat intake, only to get fatter than ever. For the first time in history, a majority of males are overweight. The previously reported relationship between higher fat consumption and resulting obesity has not been proven by scientific studies. Previously reported associations between higher fat consumption and breast cancer have been refuted. A 14-year study of nearly 89,000 women found no evidence that a high-fat diet promotes breast cancer or that a low-fat diet protects against it. Women who ate the least fat appeared to have a 15 percent higher rate of breast cancer. (Journal of the American Medical Association 3/10/99) The low fat/low cholesterol diet is ineffective. Some scientists now think that the low-fat/high carbohydrate diets are actually making us fat.

ଓଷ୍ଠଓଷ୍ଠ

WHAT ARE CARBOHYDRATES?

Your parents and grandparents probably called them starches.

All carbohydrates, whether they are in the form of rice dishes (complex carbohydrates) or a chocolate bar (simple carbohydrates), turn into glucose (blood sugar) once they enter the bloodstream. The body doesn't discriminate - - sugar is sugar. If you consume more carbohydrates than you need, your blood sugar levels will increase, triggering your pancreas to release insulin.

 CRCRCRCR

Carbohydrates are in classified in the two groups below with some examples given.

Carbohydrates	
Simple Carbohydrates	Complex Carbohydrates
Sugar	Breads
Milk	Beans
Fruit	Pastas
Juices	Potatoes
Sodas	Grains (rice, wheat,...)
Most snack foods	
Desserts	

Insulin is the "carbo squad" it controls where blood sugar is stored. Insulin is a hormone whose purpose is to convert glucose to glycogen (the stored form of sugar), which is typically stored in the liver. When needed, the glycogen can be converted back to glucose, and used as

Chapter XII - Page 279

energy. When you take in carbohydrates through the food you eat, some are used immediately for energy, and some are stored as glycogen. Since only 2,000 calories can be stored as glycogen in your body, the excess is stored as fat. Insulin also prevents existing fat from coming out of storage for use as energy since your body is getting all the energy it needs from the excess carbohydrates in the food plan most of us are following, i.e. high carbohydrate, low fat.

The interesting thing about insulin is that once you eat carbohydrates and after the insulin has finished it's job of storing the carbohydrates, it doesn't sit dormant waiting for more work; it sends an urgent signal to the brain creating false hunger pains. Naturally, you eat more to satisfy your "hunger" and the vicious cycle is repeated. With each dose of carbohydrates you produce more and more insulin causing the hunger to get worse over time. It is very important to know that as one ages cells become insulin resistant. Increased levels of insulin are required to do the same task. Unfortunately, increased levels of insulin are also related to a host of illnesses, including high blood pressure, heart disease, obesity, elevated cholesterol, hypoglycemia and diabetes.

Hypoglycemia occurs when there is too little sugar in the blood to fuel the body. It causes the dropping of blood sugar levels which can cause fatigue and symptoms like shakiness, difficulty concentrating, cold sweats, and intense hunger 1-3 hours after eating a high-carbohydrate meal, (i.e. pasta, bread, pizza, sandwiches, desserts, potatoes, and sodas). This is the normal physiologic reaction to eating a concentrated source of carbohydrates without a balance of protein or fat.

Today's health conscious society is told that fat is the cause of heart disease, cancer, and obesity. Experts are placing the blame on fat consumption. Yet, many scientists are beginning to implicate high insulin levels. They say that high fat consumption does NOT cause heart disease or high cholesterol, but that over production of insulin, or the body's resistance to insulin, causes the body to do the wrong things with the fat you eat. The arguments are very compelling and certainly should be taken into consideration.

ෲcෲcෲ

How to Lower Your Insulin Level

Simply restrict your intake of carbohydrates. It sounds simple, and it is. You can eat most vegetables, fish, fowl, meat, tofu, soy meats, tofu cheeses, low carb vegetarian burgers (many varieties), eggs, and cheeses. Since there are few carbohydrates being consumed, your body will actually burn fat for energy. It's important to remember that when on a low-carbohydrate lifestyle, you must keep your calories up so that your body does not believe it is starving. Then your body will begin to convert your fat into glucose for fuel and energy. This process will cause your insulin levels to drop and you will begin to lose weight.

 C3CRC3CR

HOW DO I BEGIN?

The answer is simple, start looking at - just one simple thing - just count carbohydrates. (I started by restricting my carbohydrate intake to 20-30 gms. a day. This will vary from individual to individual.) You don't routinely eat: bread, fruit, you don't eat routinely anything made from grains, certain vegetables, you don't drink any sugar drinks (rediscover water) and you stay away from any candy or cake.

SO WHAT CAN I EAT?

As mentioned before, you can eat most veggies, fish, fowl, meat, tofu, soy meats, tofu cheeses, eggs, and cheeses. Then I investigated the different veggie burgers and it turns out there is a tremendous variety in the carbohydrate content. Read Labels!! There is a large variance even within the realm of vegetarian burgers, some are high carbohydrate and some are low. There are outstanding books on low carbohydrate lifestyle, see References.

C3CRC3CR

How To Start

See your physician. Have your blood levels measured for cholesterol, HDL and triglycerides. Go on the Internet to our web page, www.homefirst.com, and surf the web sites which explain the low carbohydrate lifestyle. Read the excellent books that are available on low carbohydrate

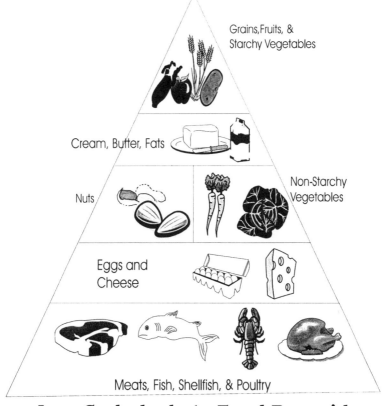

Low Carbohydrate Food Pyramid

lifestyle. Buy a carbohydrate counter book. Go to the grocery stores and read the labels. Go to an internet chat room on low carbohydrate lifestyle. You will be amazed how easy this can be. In most people, after a few weeks all the cravings for candy, soft drinks, sweets, etc. will be gone.

CRCRCRCR

REFERENCES

Atkins, Robert C. M.D., <u>New Diet Revolution</u>, Avon Books.

Atkins, Robert C., M.D., <u>Dr. Atkins' *New Carbohydrate Gram Counter*</u>, M. Evans & Co. Inc.

Borushek, Allan, <u>The Doctor's Pocket Calorie FAT & Carbohydrate Counter</u>, Family Health Publications.

Podell, Richard N. M.D., and Proctor, William, <u>The G-index Diet,</u> Warner Books.

Sears, Barry Ph.D., <u>Enter the Zone</u>, Regan Books, Harper Collins

Somers, Suzanne, <u>Get Skinny on Fabulous Food</u>, Crown, Random House.

Stewart, H Leighton, Betha, Morrison, C., Andrews, Sam S., Brennan, Ralph O., Balart, Luis A., <u>Sugar Busters</u>, Ballentine Books, 1998.

<u>www.homefirst.com</u>

EPILOGUE

Falsus in uno, falsus in omnibus.
Untrue in one thing, untrue in
everything.

Latin Expression

20th Century medicine has been shown to be false in many of its assumptions and it has held physicians with non-interventionist philosophies to a higher standard than interventionist physicians. The unscientific thinking of "I think therefore I believe" has replaced scientific evidence based decision making. How can we have trust in a medical system which has been shown to be untrue in some of its practice? The answer is with great scepticism. Let us pray that scientific reason will prevail and the motto for the 21st Century will become **"The scientific evidence points in that direction, therefore I believe".**

Homefirst® Health Services provides a full range of services in family health care in the greater Chicago metropolitan area with six medical centers - 847/679-8336 or www.homefirst.com. Our group of doctors, nurses, and certified nurse midwives dedicate themselves to providing the highest quality of health care while maintaining personalized care for each patient and family. We encourage patient involvement in the many decisions made regarding their health care.

Our care begins many times before life itself. Many couples will come to Homefirst® for pre-conception counseling. We encourage health habits that maximize the greatest chance in conceiving, maintaining a healthy pregnancy, and giving birth with the greatest efficiency and personal reward. We promote the most natural way to labor and give birth, thus avoiding unnecessary medical interventions and where the goal of an uncomplicated delivery is most likely to occur. In addition, we offer state of the art obstetrical and neonatal care if the situation calls for it. This obstetrical system has attained the highest rates of successful vaginal births and has shown that women can safely give birth at home and reap the many benefits in doing so, including a joyful and rewarding experience.

The care of the family continues after the baby is born. Breastfeeding is promoted as the foundation to maintaining the health of the newborn. It is unsurpassed in giving the baby proper nutrition. In addition, mother's milk is a source of countless other health benefits including prevention of respiratory infections, gastrointestinal illness, metabolic illness and allergies. Breast milk also contains neuropeptides which have been shown to promote brain development. Because of these advantages, Homefirst® has many resources to support the nursing relationship. Many of our nurses and receptionists are LaLeche League leaders. We also have certified lactation consultants to address the more challenging and technical problems the mother may experience.

Homefirst® also provides a full range of pediatric services as well as women's and men's health care. We continue to emphasize the philosophy of minimal use of drugs and surgery and maximal patient involvement in maintaining good health for everyone. We promote an integrative evidence based approach to managing illness. The majority of health problems are taken care of by our medical staff. When necessary, we provide referrals to a wide variety of consultants which include practitioners in alternative approaches to medicine as well as conventional medical specialists.

It has been an honor and a privilege to serve families for over 27 years, to deliver more than 14,000 babies at home and serve over 60,000 mothers, fathers, children and extended family members. Our greatest pleasure has been to provide the opportunity for our patients to grow and enrich their lives with the knowledge they are taking charge over their own health and maximizing their greatest health potential.

About the Author

DR. MAYER EISENSTEIN

Dr. Mayer Eisenstein is a graduate of the University of Illinois Medical School, the Medical College of Wisconsin School of Public Health, and the John Marshall Law School.

Since 1973 he has been in private medical practice and is currently the Medical Director of Homefirst® Health Services, the largest physician attended home birth service in the country. In his 27 years in medicine, he and his practice have delivered over 14,000 babies at home, as well as cared for over 60,000 parents, grandparents and children. Now, Dr. Eisenstein and his practice are delivering second generation babies for women who themselves were born at home with his practice.

He is Board Certified by the National Board of Medical Examiners, American Board of Public Health and Preventive Medicine, and the American Board of Quality Assurance and Utilization Review Physicians. He is a member of the National Honor Society. He is a recipient of the Howard Fellowship, Health Professional Scholarship, University of Illinois School of Medicine Scholarship, and is a member of the Dean's List at John Marshall Law School.

He is on the Professional Board of the Family Life League, Council for the Jewish Elderly, Task Force Council on Education for Public Health - Medical College of Wisconsin, and on the Editorial Board for "Child and Family Magazine". He is the author of the award winning book *Give Birth at Home With The Home Court Advantage*, as well as the editor for the "Family Health Forum" newsletter. His medical film "Primum Non Nocere" (Above All Do No Harm), a documentary on home birth, was an award winner at the Chicago Film Festival in 1987.

Some of his guest appearances include: the "Phil Donahue Show", "Milt Rosenberg Show", "Today in Chicago", "Ask the Expert", "Daybreak", "Oprah Winfrey Show", "Ed Schwartz Radio Show". "WMAQ TV news 'Unnecessary Hysterectomy'", "Chicago Fox TV News - 'Immunizations - Are They Necessary'", CBC Newsworld Canada - "Are Mass Immunizations Necessary".

Since 1987, his weekly radio show "Family Health Forum", has aired in the Chicagoland area. In September 1998 "Family Health Forum" became nationally syndicated. In the live call-in format, all listener's comments, questions or medical experiences are welcome by Dr. Eisenstein.

Dr. Eisenstein's philosophy comes from his years in medicine, combined with his years as a husband, father, and grandfather (he has six children and six grandchildren).